MW00848684

A
RUSSIAN
HERBAL

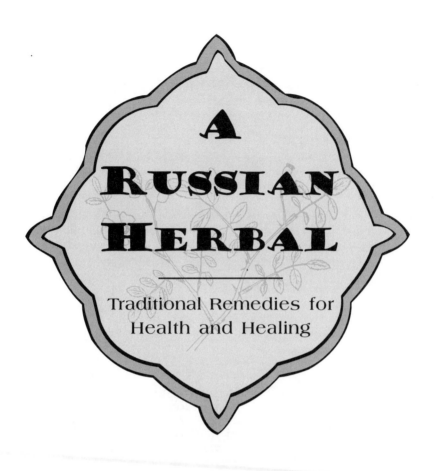

A RUSSIAN HERBAL

Traditional Remedies for
Health and Healing

IGOR VILEVICH ZEVIN
WITH NATHANIEL ALTMAN
AND LILIA VASILEVNA ZEVIN

Illustrations by Igor Vilevich Zevin

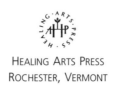

HEALING ARTS PRESS
ROCHESTER, VERMONT

Healing Arts Press
One Park Street
Rochester, Vermont 05767
www.gotoit.com

Copyright © 1997 by Igor Vilevich Zevin, Nathaniel Altman, and Lilia Vasilevna Zevin
Illustrations copyright © 1997 by Igor Vilevich Zevin

All rights reserved. No part of this book may be reproduced or utilized in any form or by
any means, electronic or mechanical, including photocopying, recording, or by any
information storage and retrieval system, without permission in writing from the publisher.

*Note to the reader: This book is intended as an informational guide. The remedies, approaches,
and techniques described herein are meant to supplement, and not to be a substitute for,
professional medical care or treatment. They should not be used to treat a serious ailment
without prior consultation with a qualified health-care professional.*

Library of Congress Cataloging-in-Publication Data

Zevin, Igor Vilevich.
A Russian herbal / by Igor Vilevich Zevin, wth Nathaniel Altman and Lilia Vasilevna Zevin
p.   cm.
Includes bibliographical references and index.
ISBN 0-89281-626-0
1. Herbs—Therapeutic use. 2. Traditional medicine—Russia.
I. Altman, Nathaniel, 1948–   . II. Zevin, Lilia Vasilevna.
III. Title.
RM666.H33Z48 1996
615'.321'0947—dc21   96-47742
CIP

Printed and bound in Canada

10 9 8 7 6 5 4 3 2 1

Type design and layout by Kristin Camp
This book was typeset in Minion with Americana and Frisky as display typefaces

Healing Arts Press is a division of Inner Traditions International

Distributed to the book trade in Canada by Publishers Group West (PGW),
Toronto, Ontario
Distributed to the health food trade in Canada by Alive Books, Toronto and Vancouver
Distributed to the book trade in the United Kingdom by Deep Books, London
Distributed to the book trade in Australia by Millennium Books, Newtown, N. S. W.
Distributed to the book trade in New Zealand by Tandem Press, Auckland
Distributed to the book trade in South Africa by Alternative Books, Randburg

CONTENTS

Part 1
Foundations   1

Introduction   2
Russian Herbalism: A Brief History   6
Collecting and Drying Herbs   13
Making Herbal Preparations   17

Part 2
A Russian Materia Medica   23

Part 3
Complex Herbal Formulas   151

The Digestive Organs   153
The Liver and Gallbladder   172
The Kidneys and Urinary Tract   178
The Cardiovascular System   185
The Respiratory System   200
The Female Reproductive System   207
The Skin and Musculoskeletal System   211
The Immune System   219
Mental and Emotional Health   224

Glossary   229
Bibliography   233
Herbal Suppliers   235
Plant Index   239
General Index   243

FOUNDATIONS

INTRODUCTION

The healing properties of medicinal plants have been recognized since the beginnings of human civilization. Specialized knowledge about herbs has been part of the folk traditions of many of the world's cultures, including the Indian, Chinese, Arabic, Tibetan, Russian, European, and Amerindian. Today, herbs are used by an estimated 86 percent of the world's population to achieve and maintain good health.

Herbs contain substances that are found nowhere else. Because most pharmaceuticals are artificially synthesized, isolated substances, the body cannot always process them as it would more natural substances. Like pharmaceuticals, herbs have a therapeutic effect on specific organ functions, body systems, and disease symptoms. Yet unlike drugs, they do not produce as many adverse reactions, especially if they are used with wisdom and common sense.

Food—including herbs—also contains a variety of micronutrients that are not generally found in nutritional supplements. Although vitamins and minerals are essential for good health, herbs are able to address specific health problems more effectively and quickly than vitamins and minerals alone.

Russia has one of the greatest traditions of herbal medicine and one that is also the least known beyond its borders. Blessed with a country with a wide variety of climates, geography, and flora, the early residents of Russia and other former Soviet republics developed a rich folk tradition of herbal healing that ranks among the most sophisticated in the world. Because of the unique geographic and geopolitical position of the former Soviet Union and the frequent invasions of Tartars, Arabs, Scandinavians, Mongolians, and Turks, which took place over the centuries, the Russian people were able to draw from the herbal traditions of many of these cultures as well as their own.

Although traditional Russian herbalism has been practiced throughout the country for centuries, medical researchers did not take a serious interest in the medicinal value of plants until early in the twentieth century. Later, after the Second World War, the State totally subsidized widespread medical research in herbalism. As a result, many of the herbs described in this book have been subjected to exhaustive laboratory research and clinical trials. Many of them have been approved by government institutions in the same manner that pharmaceutical drugs are tested and approved for their safety and effectiveness in treating human diseases, and research continues in many parts of the Federation.

Although modern Western (allopathic) medicine is practiced throughout the former Soviet republics, nearly every medical school offers courses on the knowledge and application of herbs. Many maintain a special research department that investigates the properties and practical application of herbal medicine and coordinates detailed clinical trials on human patients. The All-Union Institute of Herbs and Aromatherapy in Moscow is perhaps the largest such center in the world. It and several other research institutes (such as the Herbal Institute of Uzbekistan and others in Tbilisi, Armenia, and Harkov) are known to medical researchers in the West. Hundreds of researchers are now in the field, interviewing traditional healers and seeking to document and verify the value of both traditional Russian herbs and the thousands of remedies made from them, both alone and in combination with other plants.

In Russia today, herbs are used as both adjuncts to and as alternatives to allopathic drugs. They are either used alone or as part of complex herbal recipes that have been developed over the years by folk herbalists, physicians, and researchers. Taken until symptoms disappear, they assist the body to heal itself. When the body is able to deal with the health problem on its own, dosage is usually reduced or stopped altogether. Herbs can also be used to help maintain good health as a refreshing relaxant or tonic or can be used as preventive therapy when the individual may be more prone to disease, such as during cold or flu season.

At the present time, about 30 percent of all medicines used in the former Soviet Union are derived from medicinal plants, which is slightly more than the approximately 25 percent derived from plants in the United States. There is also a large body of scientific data based on both early Russian herbal traditions and the more recent findings of modern Soviet scientists. However, because of a past lack of interest in the West, as well as language and political barriers, most of this knowledge has not spread outside the country until now.

A Russian Herbal is the first book published in the West that reveals both the ancient traditions of herbal medicine in the former Soviet Union and their modern scientific applications today. Drawn from a wealth of traditional knowledge (both from written and oral sources), this book not only examines the best-known Russian herbs, their folkways, properties, and uses but also offers simple and clear recipes for using the herbs for specific health problems in ways that have been tested and proved safe and effective by Russian medical research, both in the laboratory and in clinical practice. While many of the herbs will be familiar to Westerners, much of the information and guidance contained in this book has never before been seen by Western readers.

In the following pages, we examine approximately one hundred different herbs that are not only found in the Russian Federation, but which can also be easily obtained in North America. We also feature an herbal "selector" for different types of health complaints. This part of the book contains approximately two hundred complex recipes using combinations of different medicinal plants that help alleviate symptoms of some forty different health problems, including specific types of heart disease, stomach and intestinal problems, skin disease, hypertension, stress, rheumatism, arthritis, respiratory problems, and tonsillitis. Special care has been taken to insure that the recipes are simple to understand, and have been proved safe and effective in Soviet medical practice.

A goal of this book is to advise the reader of any herb that Russian scientists have found to contain poisonous compounds. Unfortunately, many herbal books and herbal preparations currently on the market still lack this information. Sometimes critics cite these poisonous substances to justify a condemnation of herbalism. They forget to mention, however, that every commercially prepared pharmaceutical drug on the market today can produce adverse side effects if not used properly.

When herbs are used according to established dosages, the chances of adverse reactions are rare. However, if you are presently taking medications, you will need to find out if the combination of an herb with a commercial drug can cause a problem. For example, echinacea is an immune booster. With some patients, it may cause adverse reactions when taken with a drug like cortisone, an immune suppressor. In general, pregnant women should be very careful about what they take into their bodies, including herbs. In the descriptions of individual herbs later on in the text, we have noted those that should not be taken by pregnant women.

People often make the mistake of expecting herbs to perform miracles or, at least, to cure them of their health problem more quickly than allopathic medicines can. In many cases (though not all), herbs act more slowly than allopathic medicines and often need to be taken for a longer period of time. One advantage is an absence of adverse side effects. In addition, the herb's natural components are easily assimilated by the human body.

Finally, remember that the information in this book is for informational purposes only. In Russia, a good part of herbal medicine is used under the guidance of a physician. Treatment of serious or chronic conditions requires the care of a medical specialist or other licensed health professional.

RUSSIAN HERBALISM:
A BRIEF HISTORY

꒰ ꗃ ꒱

We all have some idea about how modern medical science came into being. We know that medicine has evolved to its present state over thousands of years, not unlike the study of mathematics or astronomy. But sometimes we forget that nonsurgical medicine has almost always been based on the use of medicinal plants. In many of the world's industrialized countries, the development of a wide variety of synthetic drugs like penicillin, tetracycline, and Valium has captured the attention of both the public and the scientific community, while interest in traditional herbal preparations has quietly slipped into the background. But recently herbal medicines have experienced a resurgence in countries like the United States, where health-care consumers are looking for low-cost, more natural preparations that are effective and have fewer adverse side effects than synthetic commercial drugs.

In many parts of the world, herbal medicine still plays a major role in healing. Even in the United States and western Europe, 25 percent of all commercial pharmaceuticals are plant based, while in Russia the number is closer to 30 percent. As botanists increase their investigations of medicinal plants from tropical rainforests and remote places in the north, such as Siberia and the tundra, this percentage is likely to increase, especially in the United States.

Although the present state of the Russian health-care system lags far behind those of the United States and western European countries, the level of medical research in Russian universities and medical centers has consistently remained at a world-class level. Like the development of nuclear weapons, rockets, and space stations, Russian medical research has always received far more emphasis than, for example, the development of consumer goods or building a viable free-market economy. The All-Union Exhibition of Achievements of National Industry in Moscow has a special pavilion devoted entirely to herbs and other medicinal plants in addition to exhibition halls devoted to spaceships, industrial technology, and agricultural machinery.

In addition to advanced study in synthetic pharmaceuticals in the former Soviet republics, ongoing research has long been undertaken in examining, evaluating, and verifying the medicinal value of herbs and the wide variety of other plants that can be found throughout the former Soviet republics. Many major medical research centers have a department specifically devoted to the study of herbs, and many Russian, Armenian, and Uzbek doctors are required to complete a course of study in herbalism before obtaining their medical degrees. Many Russian hospitals create herbal preparations in their pharmacies to give to patients, and herbs are widely available commercially throughout Russia and other former Soviet republics.

The history of herbalism traces its roots to the dawn of human existence. Like a tree with branches representing the world's civilizations, the branches of herbalism reflect the cultures from where they came. Many of the earliest uses of herbs to treat disease were a result of trial and error—tribal healers or shamans using different plants in a haphazard fashion to treat a wide variety of health complaints. Over many generations, this trial-and-error approach gradually evolved into folk-healing traditions based on both the availability of the plants and the ever-changing needs of the population. As a result, Native Americans developed their own herbal tradition, while the Chinese, Egyptians, Indians, and Tibetans developed theirs. In the dense forests and rich meadows of what is now Russia, members of the Skif and Clavac tribes made their herbal preparations from the extraordinary variety of flowers, trees, and other plants that were found there.

At the present time we have five major developed branches of herbalism: European, Asian-Arabic, Chinese, Indian, and Russian. Many other traditions were significantly altered by invasions from other cultures. Native American herbalism, for example, was close to extinction after the European settlement of North America because many of the Europeans brought their own healing tradition with them. At the same time, the whites embarked on a genocidal campaign to subjugate and exterminate the Native Americans. This included outlawing many of their traditional healing practices of which herbalism was a major part. As the development of Western allopathic medicine grew in the late 1900s, traditional, indigenous methods of healing became less valued, even among Native Americans themselves. European science showed little interest in native herbal healing, and few herbs were ever studied in a scientific manner. Although many native herbal traditions remain, mostly passed on from generation to generation, what exists today is primarily a mixture of both European and Amerindian traditions. Of course, few of the five major herbal schools were ever completely isolated, since traders and military invaders brought their herbal traditions with them. However, they were able to remain more faithful to their original form than others.

Each branch or tradition of herbalism can be divided into two subtraditions: folk-herbalism, an oral tradition passed on from generation to generation, and the "official" tradition, which is based more on scientific investigation. Originally, these two subbranches were one and the same, but the development of the written word began to divide them. The evolution of these traditions varied from culture to culture. In ancient Greece, physicians like Hippocrates, Galen, and Diascorides wrote extensively on the medicinal value of herbs, many of which, incidentally, were found in the former Soviet republic of Georgia, known then as "the magic herbal garden." Although official Russian herbal medicine came from these Grecian roots, it continued to evolve through the old word-of-mouth tradition as well.

When the early Romans conquered much of Europe, they brought their medical literature along with them. After the Roman Empire collapsed, the tribal peoples that succeeded them seized these herbals and medical texts. Over the centuries, many of these books were translated into local languages. As the many small European states became governed by more central authorities, the old oral herbal traditions (which were often fragmented and never organized) slowly lost favor. Gradually, herbalists began to place more trust in the written word than in the folk traditions. In addition, many practices were banned by the church, and many wise women (often considered to be "witches") were persecuted and even killed for applying their ancient herbal and other healing traditions. By the eighteenth century, folk healing in Europe was almost completely replaced by official medicine.

In what is now Russia, the old folk-healing tradition existed independently until the tenth century, when herbal and medical literature was first introduced. At this time, a number of Greek herbals found their way into Russia and were eventually translated into the Russian language. Unlike herbal practice in other countries, however, the Russian herbal tradition was strong and well established. Some of the new translations of herbal books, in fact, were revised to include many aspects of folk healing. And because the country was larger, more isolated, and less centrally run than other European states, it was far more difficult to introduce new ideas from Greece and Rome than in many parts of western Europe.

The long evolution of Russian herbalism also set it apart from other traditions. In addition, Russia's enormous size, different soils, and varied topography and climates favored the growth of an extensive number of herbs, trees, and other plants. This led to active interest in locally grown plants, which stimulated serious study by traditional healers and early official physicians alike.

Recently, an old chronicle was found that dates from the thirteenth century. It mentions that in the old city of Novgorod, Russian herbalists discovered the properties of the mold that eventually led to the development of penicillin in England some seven centuries later. The chronicle told how Russian herbalists (called "knowledgists") were able to cure infected wounds with "banya's mold." This example gives a good idea of the level of Russian folk medicine at that time. It is easy to understand why Russian herbalism, developed over the centuries in isolation, has evolved to the high level it enjoys today.

From the thirteenth to sixteenth centuries, European herbalism continued to develop, incorporating the old knowledge found in Greek and Roman texts. However, these developments were rarely shared with the Russians, as many of the political and cultural links between Russia and Europe were severed during that time. In the mid-thirteenth century, Tartars and Mongolians from the East invaded Russia and occupied it for over three hundred years. They brought their own herbal traditions, which Russian herbalists began studying and eventually incorporated into their healing practices.

During the fifteenth and sixteenth centuries, the Russian empire expanded as Russian troops began capturing surrounding lands and peoples. As a result, the Asian-Arabic herbal system became known to Russian herbalists belonging to both the official and folk traditions. Because Russia now counted among her neighbors countries in western Europe and Asia, Russian herbalists were able to study and compare the herbal traditions of both the East and the West with their own. The ability of the Russians to study and adopt the best features of both traditions led to the development of the unique features and advantages of the Russian herbal system.

The self-imposed isolation of China kept it from experiencing many of the scientific developments of the eighteenth and nineteenth centuries when many medical discoveries were made by Western researchers. By contrast, many of these developments were known in Russia, which at that time enjoyed close economic, political, and cultural ties with the rest of Europe. These connections were so close that at one time the predominant language of the Russian aristocracy was French rather than Russian.

Although the Russian aristocracy living in cities had ready access to modern European medical achievements, the common people still used their traditional folk medicine, which was almost completely forgotten in the rest of Europe. This lack of access to modern medicine was compounded by Russia's size, as well as poor transportation and communication links in the countryside. Because even modern physicians found it difficult to have access to modern pharmaceuticals, which were easily obtainable in large cities, they tended to focus their attention on the old and established Russian healing folkways. They also used traditional medicines as the focus for their research and published their findings in early Russian medical journals. In the beginning of the nineteenth century, one such researcher, A. T. Bolotov, published a total of nearly five hundred articles about the medicinal value of herbs.

During the nineteenth century, Professor V. M. Ambodisk-Maksimovich wrote the multivolume work *Physician's Wording*, which contained much valuable information about herbs. Works on herbalism by professors of the Russian universities, such as Ioann Georgovich Gmelin (1709–1755), Peotr Simonovich Pallas (1741–1811), and Ivan Ivanovich Lepehin (1740–1802), revealed both a thorough grounding in both modern European medicine and Russian folk-herbal tradition. In contrast, European physicians had completely forgotten about the herbal folkways that once predominated in their countries, while traditional Chinese healers had almost no awareness of the medical developments in the West. Russian doctors were unique because they knew of both their own folk-herbal traditions and modern Western medicine. This later became a defining feature of modern Russian medicine as practiced today.

By the early twentieth century, Russian scientists had developed much original material about herbs that could have been of tremendous value to physicians in other parts of the world, especially those with a geography and climate similar to those of Russia. However, after the October Revolution in 1917, Russia became closed off from the rest of the world, and this information was never shared.

Although the revolution brought about profound political, social, and economic changes throughout what had become the Soviet Union, the government did not discard Russian medicine and herbalism. In fact, the State devoted considerable attention and money to research about traditional folk healing and herbal medicine. While herbalism has been completely ignored in medical schools in the United States, nearly all Russian medical schools and universities include herbal studies in major courses. In a sense, the study of herbalism and folk healing became a type of state-run industry in the former Soviet Union. Research was carried out at special academic research institutes, and every college of pharmacy established a department exclusively devoted to the study of medicinal plants. The All-Union Institute of Herbs and Aromatherapy is perhaps the largest herbal research center in the world and is best known in the West as the agency responsible for the ongoing preservation and care of Lenin's mortal remains. Herbal institutes in Armenia, Azerbadjan, Tbilisi, and Harkov, along with the Herbal Institute of the Uzbekistan Academy, are among the best of all the former Soviet Republics. Although in recent years the majority of research monies have been given to institutes developing synthetic medicines as in the West, the work done at these special institutes has long played an important role in the development of contemporary Russian medicine. In no other country have herbs been studied so extensively using contemporary research methods with modern scientific equipment.

Russian academic herbalism began developing over fifty years ago. Before that time, medical research focused on chemical and synthetic drugs as in the West. However, when a group of antibiotics was successfully extracted from fungi and other mold-producing substances in a Russian laboratory, scientific interest in fungi and other plants grew. At about the same time, the discovery of old Russian chronicles revealed that medical discoveries related to fungi that had taken place seven hundred years before led medical researchers to campaign more aggressively for more funding to study fungi and other natural medicinals. It was also realized that many herbal and other natural remedies were the product of hundreds of years of clinical research and that their properties and side effects were quite well known. In contrast, many of the synthetically produced, chemically based medicines of the time had only been used clinically for decades at the most, and their full range of side effects was not thoroughly documented. Physicians were concerned about these negative side effects. As a result, Russian medical research focused on both modern and folk approaches to healing rather than just one.

In one approach, Russian scientists isolated one or more of the medicinal properties of a single herb or fungus in the laboratory (and possibly enhanced them chemically) to create new medications that were often more powerful than the original plant. This approach eventually led to the development of a number of new herb-based medicines as well as to the creation of synthetic pharmaceuticals that duplicated the active medicinal element in the original plant or fungus. However, not all these efforts were successful. Scientists found that the herb itself with its unique combination of chemical components was often more effective than the chemical derivatives alone. As a result, medical science also focused on the medicinal value of the herbs themselves and how they could best be incorporated into medical practice.

For example, it was found that the fruits of dog rose (rose hips) contain not only vitamin C, but also beta-carotene, tannin, vitamins B_2, K, and P, as well as sugar and a number of valuable trace elements. Combined, these elements make up a fruit with powerful medicinal properties that could not be easily (let alone inexpensively) duplicated in a laboratory.

In addition, many medicinal plants contained living cells that could be more easily incorporated into the human body than the components of synthetic drugs. Human and plant cells share many features in common, not only structurally but also in the biochemical processes that occur when they are combined. That may be one reason why even plants containing poisonous substances, such as wormwood, are often tolerated by the human body in small amounts and can even prove beneficial for health.

When we consider the value of herbs and other natural medicinals, we need to remember that the evolution of plants and animals has been closely linked throughout history. Animals cannot build their bodies with nonorganic mineral substances and must eat plants either directly or indirectly via meat and other animal products. As a result, animals have adapted to consuming plants and have built their bodies with plant substances. This direct and intimate link has created a close connection between the chemical structure of plants and animals. For this reason, different plant substances can have a profound effect on the various organs and tissues of the human body.

Scientists are continuing to learn about the many unique and subtle processes that take place in the living cell. It may take another hundred years for future generations of scientists to understand fully these complex and delicate processes. In the meantime, the laboratory of nature is constantly creating miracles every day—not in a sterile laboratory with controlled temperature, filtered air, and machines working under high pressure, but in an environment with varied temperatures, germs, fungi, and normal atmospheric pressure. While laboratory research is important and must continue, getting back to "nature's medicine chest" is finally being recognized to be of immediate and lasting value. At least one major drug company in the United States is researching medicinal plants in the Costa Rican rainforest, while a new company, Shaman Pharmaceuticals, is completely devoted to formulating drugs from traditional herbal preparations.

While the science of synthetic medicine moves ahead, perhaps Western scientists and healers will take another look at the value of herbs and partake of the highly developed and unique Russian herbal medical tradition largely unknown in the West.

COLLECTING AND DRYING HERBS

❦

Many people discover that searching for and collecting their own medicinal herbs in the fields and forests can be a highly rewarding experience. On the following pages, we will offer general guidelines for herb collecting and drying according to the Russian herbal tradition.

Collecting Herbs

When we speak of herbs, we usually mean the leaves, stems, and flowers. With some herbs, such as everlasting, the roots are included as well.

In Russia, herbalists collect the stems at the time of blossoming, before the seeds or fruit are mature. Generally speaking, the herb is cut with a sharp knife at the base of the plant, just above ground level. Before cutting, the herb should be examined carefully to make sure that it contains no brownish or yellowing areas, and is free from foreign particles.

Place the entire herb in a thin layer on clean cloth. Allow to dry in the open air or in a clean, well-ventilated room. Russians often devote a room in a barn for this purpose; rooms containing fiberglass insulation are usually avoided. As a general rule, the ideal temperature for drying herbs is between 104 and 128 degrees Farenheit (°F) (38 and 53 degrees Celsius [°C]), which approximates the temperature in the sun during the summer, or under strong fluorescent lighting. Some herbs that contain ether oil should be dried at lower temperatures, ranging from 86 to 100°F (30 to 38°C).

With some herbs (such as thyme, wild marjoram, and St. Johnswort), the thick stems are removed after drying. The dried herb should consist of flowers, leaves, and short thin stems and should retain the plant's original taste, smell, and color.

Collecting Flowers

In general, flowers should be collected while in full blossom. The primary exceptions are chamomile flowers and everlasting flowers, which are collected while the flower is blossoming. Pick the flowers by hand or remove carefully with a sharp knife.

Make sure that the flowers you select are free of defects (such as dead petals or brown edges) and are similar to flowers on neighboring plants of the same species. The flowers should also be free from foreign matter such as insect eggs.

Dry the flowers in a well-ventilated room. Spread them in a thin layer on a paper towel or brown wrapping paper. The dried flowers should be whole and retain the natural color and aroma of the fresh flowers.

Collecting Leaves

Leaves can be collected right before and during the time of blossoming. Carefully remove leaves from the plant, making sure that you do not remove more than a third of the plant's leaves. Make sure that the collected leaves are free from any defects, such as insect bites, discoloration, or the presence of growths or fungi. Generally speaking, leaves should be whole and of uniform color and aroma. Place the leaves on a clean, dry kitchen towel in a well-ventilated room.

Collecting Roots

For the most part, roots and rootstocks are best collected in the fall when the plant is preparing itself for winter. Some roots, however, are collected during the early spring when the plant contains more medicinal substances than it does in the fall.

The roots are gently dug up with a small spade or shovel. They are then washed in running water to remove soil and other extraneous matter. The roots of certain plants (such as licorice) are not washed, because washing reduces their medicinal potency. Some roots should be shorn of their tiny accessory roots.

Large roots are usually sliced into two or three thin pieces to speed up the drying process and to prevent the formation of molds. Like other parts of the herb, roots should be dried in a well-ventilated room and should maintain their original smell, taste, and color.

Collecting Berries

Berries or fruits should be ripe at the time of collection. Some plants drop their fruits before they are ripe, so it is best to collect these fruits before they are fully ripened. The best time for collection is in the mornings or evenings. With some plants, the branches that hold the fruits are cut with a sharp knife and tied into small bundles for drying. After drying, the fruits are removed from the branches and cleaned.

Juicy fruits (such as raspberries) are collected when they are ripe. The best time for harvesting is on dry, cloudy days or in the mornings or evenings on hot days. Bruised or imperfect fruits should not be used for medicinal purposes.

Make sure that all foreign particles, including pieces of stems or leaves as well as unripened fruits, are removed before drying. Place the berries on a piece of clean, thick paper, a clean, dry cloth, or cloth stretched on a frame. Russian collective farms often have special drying machines for berries and herbs. The ideal temperature for drying berries is between 75 and 90°F (25 to 32°C) at low humidity.

After drying, carefully examine the berries for defects and clean them of foreign particles. Though dry, the berries should possess their natural smell, taste, and color. Dark, moldy berries or berries with dry spots should be composted.

Generally speaking, seeds are collected and dried in a similar manner. However, the exact method will vary with the type of plant.

Collecting Buds

It is better to collect buds in the spring when they are swelling, but not when they are still green. Birch buds can be collected earlier, usually from mid-February through the first week in March. Pine buds are collected from October through May. Cut the tip of the stem no longer than 1¼ inches. Pine and birch buds should be dried in a cool, well-ventilated room to prevent blossoming. Remember to harvest only small amounts from each tree so that the tree can reproduce properly.

Collecting Bark

In Russia, herbalists usually collect bark in early spring when the sap begins flowing through the tree. To find out if the sap is flowing, make a small cut through the bark of the tree or bush; a small amount of sap will soon appear. At this time it is easy to remove the bark. Harvest the bark from young branches of trees between three and four years of age. Cut two rings on a branch, 10 to 12 inches apart, with a sharp knife. Make two more cuts along the length of the branch, connecting the two ring cuts. Pull up at one end, and the bark will peel off the tree.

Be sure the bark is thoroughly cleaned (a firm-bristled toothbrush can be used) and free of any foreign matter. Any rotted areas should be discarded. Upon returning home, place the bark on a dry cloth in the open air with the pieces lying apart from each other. After drying, inspect the bark and be sure that it is free of defects or discoloration.

The process of collecting and drying some herbs will differ from the general guidelines described here. These exceptions will be noted in the herb descriptions later on.

Although many readers will decide to purchase their herbs directly from herbal suppliers (a listing of some of them is included in the resources section), I encourage readers to collect their own herbs in the field or grow them in their gardens.

If at all possible, it is best to venture into the countryside to collect herbs yourself. This should be done with the aid of a good field guide to native plants that contains color drawings or photographs of the featured plants. However, the best way is to search for herbs with an experienced herbalist or person with a good knowledge of plants. From my own experience as a young man learning about herbs in Byelorussia (now Belarus), I appreciated having a more knowledgeable person point out species of herbs to me when I visited fields, forests, and botanical gardens in my search for herbal knowledge.

Making Herbal
Preparations

Methods of making herbal preparations depend on several factors: the ability of the herbal substance to dissolve in cold or hot water, the type and character of the herb, and the diseases or other health problems the herb is to be used for. It can also depend on the personal taste of the patient.

Russian herbalists usually recommend adding 1 tablespoon of fresh herb or roots to 1 cup of water. A similar ratio is recommended when dried, crushed herbs are used. Most herbalists use dried herbs, which are gathered, dried, and stored until they are needed. This is why many of the recipes in this book call for dried herbs. Generally speaking, the dried herbs are crushed just before making an herbal preparation and are measured in their crushed state. If store-bought herbal teabags are used, I recommend two teabags per 1½ cups (375 ml) of water. However, this should not be a rule, since we need to consider the type of herb and the way it is to be used.

Infusions

Nearly all plants are water soluble, which means that their chemical and medicinal compounds can be dissolved in water. Hot infusions are made by pouring boiling water over the fresh or dried herb and letting it steep for a specific amount of time, usually fifteen minutes or more. Most herb teas are prepared as hot infusions, many of which are described later in this book.

Herbs whose medicinal value is destroyed by heat are prepared as cold infusions. Generally speaking, infusions work best with the soft, above-ground parts of plants, such as the flowers, leaves, and soft fruits.

Most infusions are taken when they are cool enough to drink. If you need to save a medicinal infusion for future use, strain the liquid, pour the infusion into a bottle, close with a tight stopper, and store in the refrigerator for up to three days. Some herbal preparations can be stored for longer periods of time, which will be noted in the text.

Many Russian herbalists consider that fresh herbs, gently crushed, are more effective than dry, although there are many herbs which should only be used when dried. When describing herbal preparations later in the text, measurements are given both by weight and by volume. Either measurement can be used for dried herbs that are gently crushed. However, if fresh herbs are used, the weight measurements are best.

Decoctions

Decoctions are made by boiling the fresh or dried herb in water for a specified amount of time to extract its medicinal value. This method is often used with the stems or roots of plants, as well as the bark of trees and certain types of dried fruits. In making a decoction, the ingredients are often finely chopped or crushed and either added to cold water and boiled or added to water that is already boiling. Although most herbs are boiled from 10 to 15 minutes, different herbs may require more or less time. The decoction is then filtered and allowed to sit until cool enough to drink.

Most decoctions are consumed like tea, but they can also be used as compresses by soaking a cloth in the decoction and applying it to affected body parts.

The Water Banya

One of the best-known methods of preparing medicinal herbs in Russia is the water *banya* or bath. It was developed by Russian herbalists, and it has generally not been known outside Russia until now.

This method is especially popular with experienced herbalists when they need to prepare complex recipes. The water banya uses steam to dissolve substances that lie deep in the plant and allows several plants to be blended without losing their individual identity. In addition, the water banya avoids burning the herbs and also helps maintain their aroma.

First, the herbalist crushes or chops the herbal material before combining it with others. Generally speaking, leaves and flowers are no longer than $1/4$ inch, while stems and bark are no larger than $1/8$ inch, and fruits, berries, and seeds are crushed or cut to sizes no larger than $1/8$ inch.

The crushed or chopped material is then placed in a pot made from ceramic, tempered glass, or stainless steel. Many herbalists prefer an enamel pot with a wide bottom and a narrow neck and a lid with a small hole. For one preparation, the pot can accommodate up to 2 tablespoons of dried herbs and 1 cup of water. The mixture should take up approximately three-fourths of the volume of the pot. Professional herbalists often use a pot that is four to five times larger than the mixture in order to prepare three to six doses at once. They usually refrigerate what they do not immediately need for future use. If the herbal formula needs to be reheated, it is usually done in a covered enamel pot over low heat.

The herbalist places a small plate upside down inside, on the bottom, of a larger pot. The smaller pot is placed on the plate. The larger pot is then filled with water so that the level is three-fourths of the depth of the smaller pot, as shown in figure 1.

Usually, boiling water is poured into both pots. The smaller pot is often of a heavier gauge than the larger pot. It is topped by a heavy lid or the lid is weighed down by a heavy object.

The water in the larger pot is boiled again over a low flame for 10 to 15 minutes. Extra water may be added every 5 minutes as it evaporates. The water in the smaller pot is boiling as well, but since it is covered, most of the

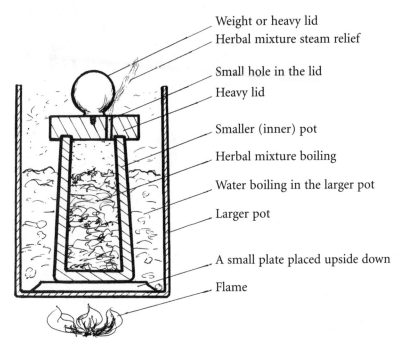

Weight or heavy lid

Herbal mixture steam relief

Small hole in the lid

Heavy lid

Smaller (inner) pot

Herbal mixture boiling

Water boiling in the larger pot

Larger pot

A small plate placed upside down

Flame

Figure 1. The Water Banya

water does not evaporate: it circulates through the pot. The smaller pot also maintains a uniform temperature. This keeps the herbs from burning and allows them to mix more easily.

After boiling for 15 minutes, the herbalist turns off the heat and lets the herbs steep for approximately 45 minutes. The smaller pot is then carefully removed and the infusion is filtered.

This is the traditional Russian method for infusing complex recipes. The water banya can also be used to make decoctions, but the boiling process continues for 30 minutes or more. In some cases, extra water is added to the small pot, since 30 minutes of boiling will cause more water to evaporate. After the boiling process is complete, herbalists allow the herbal mixture to steep for 10 minutes before the decoction is strained.

As can be imagined, assembling the equipment for the water banya takes some time, and the actual process requires practice to make it successful. However, using this method will enhance the medicinal value of the recipes, so it is well worth the effort.

The Thermos Method

A simpler alternative to the water banya employs a thermos bottle in making complex herbal formulas. This method involves adding 1 table-spoon of the herbal mixture to 1 cup or so of water, bringing the water to a boil, and then simmering the decoction for several minutes. The liquid is then poured into a thermos bottle, where it is sealed and allowed to steep for several hours or more, depending on the recipe. The liquid is then strained and used.

Some Russian herbalists use a thermos bottle that can be heated in a special oven while it is steeping. Since this may not be easily available here in the West, we recommend reheating the decoction to a comfortable drinking temperature.

Tinctures

Tinctures are concentrated herbal preparations made with alcohol. They are made by steeping 2 to 4 ounces (57 to 113 g) of herbs in alcohol for a period of two weeks. Use a glass bottle with a tight lid. The bottle should be kept at room temperature and shaken once a day. Strain the tincture before using.

Herbalists recommend using at least 90-proof spirits for most tinctures. In Russia, vodka is commonly used for this purpose, although other types of spirits can be used as well. One advantage that tinctures have over decoctions and infusions is that they have a longer shelf life: the alcohol acts as a preservative. Generally speaking, tinctures are very concentrated, so only a few drops need be used at a time.

Juices

Fresh herbal juices can be used externally or internally to treat a variety of conditions. To prepare a basic juice, wash freshly picked aerial parts in cold water and rinse in hot water. Process the herb in a food grinder and strain the resulting pulp in cheesecloth, squeezing well to extract as much of the juice as possible. Dilute with 2 parts of water for every 1 part of juice. Heat to boiling and then simmer gently for 1 or 2 minutes. Remove from heat and allow to cool to a comfortable temperature before using. The juice can be stored in the refrigerator in a tightly closed container for a week.

A Russian
Materia Medica

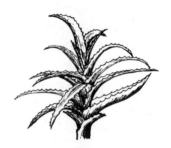

ALOE
Botanical name: *Aloe vera.*
Family: Liliaceae.

Although aloe is not native to Russia, it has long been studied and used in both official and traditional Russian herbal medicine. Preparations of aloe were first processed in the 1900s by the famous Russian academician V. P. Filatov to heal human tissues. He proved that aloe's biogenical stimulators exert a strong influence on the human organism. His preparations were used primarily in treating eye problems.

Although native to desert areas, aloe vera is a good indoor plant, requiring full sun or light shade. Russians have grown aloe in their homes since the 1930s and use it for treating cuts, scrapes, minor burns, cold sores, sunburn, and other types of skin inflammation. They cut off a leaf and split it into two parts, applying the gel from the center of the leaf to the wound. Sometimes a bandage is placed over both the leaf and the wound, but aloe works best when the skin is exposed to the open air.

Parts used: Leaves.

Actions: Antibacterial, antiseptic, emollient, laxative, moisturizer, purgative, vulnerary.

Medicinal virtues: The aloe vera plant contains salicylate, which is the same pain-killing and anti-inflammatory compound found in aspirin. Used externally, aloe breaks down the dead tissue in a wound and helps regenerate new tissue. It has been used to treat radiation burns and frostbite. Russian dermatologists, ophthalmologists, and gynecologists use aloe to treat burns, wounds, boils, and other skin conditions and irritations, including sunburn, wrinkles, and insect bites.

Taken internally, fresh juice is used to treat stomach and intestinal ulcers, diseases of the digestive tract, and gastric hyperacidity. It is also used in Russian official medicine to stimulate appetite. Dr. Filatov has used an aloe extract to stimulate the body's immune system when treating ulcers and other debilitating conditions, as well as to treat problems in the respiratory system.

Aloe juice is also a strong laxative. For this reason it is better to drink the juice in the morning on an empty stomach (the laxative action starts after

8 to 10 hours). However, using aloe internally has been linked with a number of adverse side effects, including hemorrhoidal and uterine bleeding. In addition, some people who are hypersensitive to aloe can develop a rash if it is taken internally.

Habitat and collection: Aloe is cultivated primarily as an indoor plant, since it does poorly when the temperature falls below 41°F (5°C). Grow in a sunny place or one with full shade. Cut the leaves from the plant when needed.

Preparation and dosage: To use aloe externally, cut open the leaf and apply the gel directly to the wound. You can also use the gel as a moisturizer on dried or chapped skin.

Fresh aloe vera gel is an excellent hair conditioner. Break open the leaf and rub the gel through your hair. Leave for 15 minutes and then shampoo thoroughly.

For internal use, aloe juice can be made by squeezing the finely chopped leaves through a piece of cheesecloth. Take 1 teaspoon (5 ml) 2 to 3 times a day before meals. Dr. Filatov suggests that you wash the leaves in water and keep them in a refrigerator for 2 weeks before preparing an extract.

You can also preserve the juice in honey. The Russian herbalist N. Kovaliova's recipe follows: Take 5$\frac{1}{4}$ ounces (150 g) of fresh leaves, being sure to trim the leaves of spines. Chop by hand. Heat 1 ounce (30 g) of honey and $\frac{1}{2}$ cup (125 ml) of water to boiling. Pour the honey over the leaves. Squeeze the mixture to make an extract and strain. Take 1 to 2 teaspoons (5 to 10 g) every morning one hour before meals.

Caution: Internal aloe preparations should be used only under the supervision of a qualified health-care professional. Taken internally, aloe vera can stimulate uterine contractions, and therefore should be avoided during pregnancy.

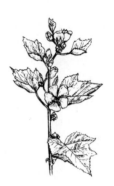

ALTHAEA

Botanical name: *Althaea officinalis.*
Family: Malvacae.
Also known as: Marshmallow, mallards,
   mortification root.

Althaea is a perennial plant that grows in the wild. It is also cultivated by herbalists throughout Russia and northern Europe. A popular Russian folktale about the healing power of althaea dates from the Mongol invasion over a thousand years ago, which was often marked by extreme and irrational cruelty. It seems that the son of a Tartar warlord had a severe cough, which no one in the village was able to heal. The father announced that he would kill one villager a day until the child was cured. The villagers were mad with grief over this terrible announcement and prepared themselves for the worst. But a local wise woman, who had an extensive knowledge of herbs, decided to help. She pulled up several althaea plants and mashed the roots. That afternoon she brought them to the warlord to give to his son and told the boy to chew the roots every few hours. By the next morning the cough was gone, and the villagers were spared their terrible fate.

Althaea has been a part of Russian, European, and Greek herbal traditions for centuries. The German emperor Karl the Great (who ruled during the seventeenth and eighteenth centuries) issued written recommendations to the citizenry to cultivate althaea in their gardens. It was also grown extensively in the gardens of Russian monasteries.

While the Russian folk tradition has always used the roots, leaves, and flowers, official Russian medicine has focused primarily on the medicinal value of the roots because the flowers and leaves do not contain as much mucilage and essential oils as the roots do.

Parts used: Flowers, leaves, roots.

Actions: Anodyne, demulcent, emollient, expectorant.

Medicinal virtues: Because althaea contains mucilage and starch, it is used to soothe the mucous layers of the body and protect them from irritation. Russian scientists have found a direct correlation between hydrochloric acid of the stomach and viscosity (stickiness) from the mucilage of althaea; when the acidity of the stomach increases, the viscosity increases as well and protects the mucous layers of the stomach. For this reason, the herb is used to treat gastritis, stomach ulcers, and irritations in the intestines and colon, such as enterocolitis.

The herb can be used to treat quinsy (an abscess due to bacterial inflammation of the tonsillar area) and jaundice. Preparations of althaea are also prescribed to treat kidney stones and to help relieve difficult urination. A cold extract of althaea is often recommended as an eyewash to relieve inflamed eyelids. It is also used as an adjunct to medication in Russia to treat pneumonia and to ease inflammation of the upper respiratory passages. An infusion of leaves and flowers makes a soothing gargle.

Habitat and collection: Althaea is found in northern Europe, Asia, and North America and tends to grow primarily in marshes, near rivers and lakes, and in damp meadows. It is best to harvest the leaves and flowers in the summer, although roots can be collected in either spring or fall. Peel the roots before using.

Preparation and dosage: To make an infusion, add 2 teaspoons (10 g) of crushed flowers or leaves (fresh or dried) to 1 cup (250 ml) of boiling water. Allow to steep for 5 minutes. Filter. Take 1/4 to 1/3 cup (62 to 100 ml) three times a day during meals.

To make a decoction, add 1 tablespoon (15 g) of chopped roots to 1 cup (250 ml) of water. Simmer the mixture on low heat for 30 minutes. Allow to cool for 10 minutes. Filter and squeeze out all remaining moisture. Take 1/3 to 1/2 cup (80 to 125 ml), either warm or hot, at mealtimes. The course of treatment can continue from 4 to 6 weeks. A cold decoction can be made by adding 2 teaspoons (10 g) of powdered root to 1 cup (250 ml) of cold water. Let stand for 8 hours. Strain. Take 2 tablespoons (30 ml) 4 to 5 times a day.

ANGELICA

Botanical name: *Angelica archangelica.*
Family: Umbelliferae.
Also known as: Garden angelica,
    European angelica. In the United States,
    Angelica atropurpurea generally resembles
    Angelica archangelica.

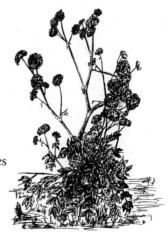

Although Russian official medicine refers to rootstocks and roots as the part of the herb recommended for collecting and medicine practice, Russian folk tradition also uses seeds and leaves. So-called angelic water made from seeds has been used by folk healers as a remedy for stomach disorders and as an antispasmodic.

Parts used: Leaves, roots, rootstocks, seeds.

Actions: Anthelmintic, antiphlogistic, appetizer, calmative, carminative, cholagogue, diaphoretic, digestive, diuretic, expectorant, nervine, sedative, sudorific, tonic.

Medicinal virtues: Preparations of angelica promote relaxation of the smooth (nonstriated) muscles of the internal organs and increase the natural secretions of the stomach and bronchial glands. Angelica also exerts a bacteriocidal effect that suppresses gastric fermentation and has a tonic influence on the cardiovascular and the central nervous systems. It increases the flow of bile into the intestines and the secretion of pancreatic juices and is a good diuretic.

Russian folk healers use angelica as a tonic to treat hysteria, epilepsy, and insomnia and as an expectorant and diaphoretic to treat diseases of the respiratory system. They also use it to treat podagra and rheumatism as well as pain in the lumbar region of the back. A decoction of leaves is used to expel intestinal worms.

Habitat and collection: Angelica is native to the European part of Russia, Belarus, Ukraine, and parts of western Siberia. It tends to grow in damp places, especially in fields near rivers, lakes, and streams. In the first year, harvest the roots during the fall; in the second year, during the spring. Dig the roots up by shovel, shake the soil off the roots, and wash them in cold water. Cut them crosswise. Dry the roots under a cover between 85 and

104°F (35 to 40°C), spreading them out in a thin layer. Store the dried roots in a closed wooden container for up to three years.

Preparation and dosage: To make an infusion, pour 1 cup (250 ml) of boiling water over 3 tablespoons (45 g) of dried roots. Cover and allow to stand for 30 minutes; then remove cover and steep for 10 minutes more. Strain. Consume ¹/₂ cup (125 ml) 2 to 3 times a day after eating. The infusion should be taken warm.

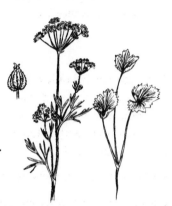

ANISE
Botanical name: *Pimpinella anisum.*
Family: Liliaceae.
Also known as: Anise plant, common anise.

Anise has been cultivated and used both as a spice and as a medicinal herb since ancient Egyptian times and is one of the first herbs accepted by Russian herbalists from the southeastern herbal traditions. Anise has been a very common herbal remedy in Russia since the beginning of the nineteenth century, when a landlord began cultivating the herb in the province of Voronez. At the present time, anise is grown on large farms throughout the northern Caucasus and Ukraine for use as both a culinary spice and herbal medicine.

It is also a major ingredient in some of the most popular over-the-counter remedies sold in Russian pharmacies.

Parts used: Seeds.

Actions: Antipyretic, antispasmodic, carminative, digestive, diuretic, expectorant, galactagogue, stimulant, stomachic, tonic.

Medicinal virtues: An aniseed infusion is used to treat inflammation of the mucous membranes of the respiratory tract and is a popular remedy for acute bronchitis, pneumonia, bronchial asthma, and whooping cough. It is also an excellent stomach remedy. It increases secretions of stomach acid and reduces nausea, flatulence, and diarrhea. Russian herbalists have long used it for relieving inflammation of the digestive tract and to promote digestion. Aniseeds also normalize the secretions of the stomach, liver, and abdominal salivary gland. It helps remove stones from the urinary tract, is used to treat vertigo and migraines, and is a recommended remedy for colic in infants. Folk herbalists recommend adding a few crushed seeds to a cup of hot milk a half hour before bedtime to promote restful sleep. Aniseeds promote the production of milk in nursing mothers who suffer from lacteal insufficiency; they also help alleviate painful menstrual cramps.

Habitat and collection: Anise grows throughout the countryside and is widely cultivated in herb gardens. Collect the seeds during August or September when the first umbels appear. Dry in the open air or in an oven heated to 122 to 140°F (50 to 60°C). You can store the dried aniseed for up to three years in a closed container.

Preparation and dosage: To make an infusion, add 1 cup (250 ml) of boiling water to 1 teaspoon (5 g) of crushed seeds. Cover and steep for 20 minutes. Strain. Take ¹/₂ cup (125 ml) 3 to 4 times a day 30 minutes before meals.

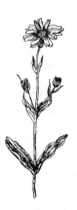

ARNICA
Botanical name: *Arnica montana.*
Family: Compositae.
Also known as: Mountain tobacco,
   wolfsbane.

In centuries past, arnica was a popular folk remedy in western Europe, where herbal manuscripts first mentioned it in the eleventh century. Russian herbalists in the western parts of the former Soviet Union (including Ukraine, Belarus, and the Karpatskie Mountains) also used the herb, but arnica was little known in the rest of the country, where it didn't grow naturally.

After complex research on the plant at several Soviet research institutions, it was decided to cultivate arnica in other regions of the country. The All-Union Institute of Herbs began planting arnica on a large scale in 1955 and soon achieved positive results in cultivating two new types that could grow in central Russia and Siberia.

Parts used: Flowers, rootstocks.

Actions: Antipyretic, cardiac, cholagogue, diaphoretic, emollient, hemostatic, sedative, tonic, vulnerary.

Medicinal virtues: An infusion made from arnica is a popular herbal remedy for a variety of heath problems. Small dosages have a tonic effect on the central nervous system, while large dosages work as a sedative and reduce stomach cramps. It is a vasodilator and has been found to reduce serum cholesterol. In cases of stenocardia, it has a cholagogue effect, and official herbalists recommend arnica for treating myocarditis, endocarditis, and cardiosclerosis. It also reduces arterial pressure and intensifies bile flow. In Russia, arnica is used in obstetrics to control uterine hemorrhage during childbirth.

In Russian folk medicine, a decoction of arnica is recommended for treating stomach problems that result from poor digestion, including ulcers, stomach spasms, and intestinal cramps. It is also an effective remedy for treating podagra and epilepsy as well as colds, influenza, and bladder problems.

When used externally, a lotion or cold wash of arnica promotes the fast healing of minor wounds, bruises, scrapes, minor burns, and frostbite. It is also prescribed for treating furuncles, carbuncles, abscesses, and trophic ulcers.

Habitat and collection: Although widely cultivated, arnica is native to mountainous areas of Russia, including the Urals and Caucasus. It is also native to other areas of Europe, Canada, and the northern United States. Arnica flowers can be collected between June and August.

Preparation and dosage: To prepare an infusion, add 1 tablespoon (15 g) of dried flowers to $^1/_2$ cup (125 ml) of hot water. Cover and allow to stand for 10 minutes. Strain. Take 3 tablespoons 3 times a day.

To make a decoction, add 1 tablespoon (15 g) of dried flowers to 1 cup (250 ml) of hot water. Bring to a boil, then lower heat and simmer for 3 to 5 minutes, stirring constantly. Cool and strain. Take 2 tablespoons (30 ml) 3 times daily before meals.

Caution: **Arnica should be taken internally only under the guidance of a qualified health-care professional. A normal course of treatment should not exceed 7 to 10 days.**

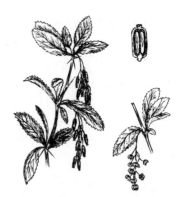

BARBERRY

Botanical name: *Berberis vulgaris.*
Family: Berberidaceae.
Also known as: Sowberry, jaundice
   berry, piperage.

The first written references to barberry date from 650 B.C.E., when the herb's "blood cleansing" properties were mentioned on an earthenware slab in the library of King Ashshiurbanipal of Assyria. Another manuscript from the sixteenth century found in the Pskov region of Russia refers to barberry's ability to cure a disease that prevented women from becoming pregnant. It was believed that Princess Xenia of Pskov used an extract made with barberry leaves to enable her to conceive an heir. In books documenting Russia's colonization of the east, references have been made to barberry's widespread growth in southern Siberia. In the 1960s Russian scientists began to study barberry for pharmaceutical use.

Parts used: Bark, fruit, leaves, roots.

Actions: Antiphlogistic, antiseptic, astringent, cholagogue, depurative, diuretic, hemostatic, hepatic, laxative, purgative, sudorific, tonic, vasodilator.

Medicinal virtues: Because the root bark contains alkaloids that promote the secretion of bile, Russian herbalists have found that a decoction of barberry root or bark is a perfect remedy for various liver and gallbladder ailments, including chronic hepatitis, gallstones, jaundice, and hepacholecystitis. A decoction of crushed roots or leaves is prescribed for stomach and duodenal ulcers. Barberry is believed to tone up the function of the gastrointestinal tract and stimulate the functions of the pancreas. Russian herbalists use a root decoction for relieving symptoms of colitis as well as for treating bladder and urinary tract infections. It's considered a very helpful remedy for overcoming morphine addiction. As a diaphoretic, a barberry root decoction is used to treat an enlarged spleen as a result of malaria.

A decoction from the berries improves circulation of the blood; it tends to dilate the blood vessels and lower blood pressure and increases blood coagulation. An infusion of barberry leaves promotes uterine contractions, which help limit menstrual bleeding. Used externally, a barberry decoction is used to treat eczema and neurodermatitis.

Habitat and collection: Barberry is a shrub that grows in rocky soil and in thickets in Europe and North America. Collect the roots and bark in either March or November. The leaves and berries can be collected in late summer.

Preparation and dosage: To make a decoction, add 1 teaspoon (5 g) of dried crushed roots to 1 cup (250 ml) of boiling water. Continue to boil for 10 minutes. Cool and strain. Take 4 tablespoons (60 ml) 4 times daily.

To prepare an infusion, add 1 teaspoon (5 g) of fresh or dried leaves to 1 cup (250 ml) of hot water. Steep for 10 minutes and then strain. Take ¹/₃ cup (80 ml) 3 times a day.

To make a vodka infusion, add 4 teaspoons (20 g) of leaves to ¹/₃ cup (80 ml) of vodka. Allow to stand in a warm place for 10 to 15 days (the liquid will be dull yellow, transparent, and have a sour taste). Take 30 to 40 drops 2 to 3 times a day for 14 to 21 days.

Caution: This herb should be avoided during pregnancy.

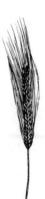

BARLEY
Botanical name: *Hordeum vulgare.*
Family: Graminaceae.

Barley is one of Russia's most important agricultural plants. The Russian Federation is the largest producer of barley in the world, and the annual harvest makes up approximately one-quarter of the world's production. As in other countries, the majority of the barley grown is used as animal feed, although it is an important source of human food and medicine as well.

An important feature of barley is its rapid growth rate: under ideal conditions, certain types of barley can be harvested only forty days after planting. In areas of northern Russia, where the growing season is very short, barley is a very important food grain. In the south, the frequency of droughts also limits the growing season, and barley is often grown during the rainy periods between droughts.

Because a limited variety of crops and other plants grow in the extreme north and south of Russia, people living in those regions made good use of the little they had. This is the main reason why they gradually learned to use barley as a medicinal plant.

Parts used: Grain.

Actions: Anthelmintic, antiphlogistic, appetizer, demulcent, diuretic, mucilaginous, nutrient, tonic.

Medicinal virtues: A decoction made from pearl barley has long been valued to help relieve diseases of the stomach and intestines. It is also used as a tonic for patients who have recently undergone abdominal surgery and is recommended for treating inflammations of the bladder and the kidneys. A barley decoction is used to relieve colds, bronchitis, and cough. Herbalists also recommend a fresh barley decoction as an anthelmintic to treat ascariasis, caused by intestinal worms.

In official dermatology, barley is used both internally and externally to treat many skin problems. Taken internally, barley malt treats a wide variety of health problems, including psoriasis, lichen planus, collagenosis, furunculosis, vitiligo, pimples, and baldness. Barley malt baths are considered effective for relieving symptoms of dermatitis, ichthyosis, and erythroderma. A poultice made from barley malt and barley flowers is used for treating mastitis, furunculosis, and other inflammatory diseases.

In folk medicine, barley is used to treat diseases of the bladder and urinary tract, as well as kidney stones and hemorrhoids. Barley is also used to relieve swelling and is believed to reduce tumors and clear jaundice. Russian folk herbalists use barley malt extract to treat diabetes. Barley mucilage is used to relieve diarrhea and pain from colitis.

Habitat and collection: Barley is cultivated throughout Europe and North America.

Preparation and dosage: To make a decoction, add 20 grains of barley to 1 cup (250 ml) of hot water. Bring to a boil, then reduce heat and simmer for 10 minutes. Take 1 to 2 tablespoons (15 to 30 ml) 4 to 6 times a day to treat diarrhea and other intestinal problems.

To prepare an infusion, soak 2 tablespoons (30 g) of barley grains in a 1-quart (1-liter) wide-mouthed jar for 12 to 16 hours. Drain off the water and cover loosely with cheesecloth or nylon netting. Keep at room temperature, and rinse twice a day. After the barley sprouts are about 1-inch long, place them on a clean cloth to dry, then run them through a food grinder. Add 2 to 3 tablespoons (30 to 40 g) of the ground barley sprouts to 1 quart (1 liter) of boiling hot water. Steep for 4 to 5 hours. Take $^1/_2$ cup (125 ml) 3 times a day.

To prepare a bath, boil 2.2 pounds (1 kg) of barley sprouts in 5 quarts to 2 gallons (5 to 8 liters) of water for 30 minutes. Strain. Add to bath water to relieve symptoms of radiculitis or arthritis.

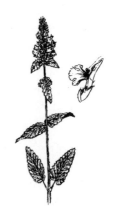

BETONY

Botanical name: *Betonica officinalis.*
Family: Labiatae.

The Russian name for this herb means "a small letter of the alphabet," suggesting that the plant resembles a fine, handwritten letter from old Russian manuscripts. Throughout the Middle Ages, betony was a popular folk remedy. It entered official medicine about a century ago when Russian doctors found it useful in treating tuberculosis. Betony is also a valuable source of various patented medications in France and Germany.

Parts used: Aerial parts.

Actions: Antihypertensive, astringent, calmative, cholagogue, digestive, diuretic, expectorant, hemostatic, purifier, sedative, stomachic, vulnerary.

Medicinal virtues: In official Russian medicine, betony is used primarily as a digestive to improve appetite, as well as for the treatment of nephritis and cystitis.

Betony is used widely as a folk remedy. A betony infusion or decoction is often prescribed for relieving inflammation of the respiratory tract, as well as for treating other lung and bronchial conditions, including asthma. Betony has the ability to thin phlegm, which makes expectoration easier and reduces coughing. Russian herbalists recommend using a betony decoction as part of a complex treatment for tuberculosis and bronchiectasis. It is also used as a hemostatic to control bleeding of the lungs.

A betony infusion is recommended for relief of gastritis due to hyperacidity, as well as for reducing pain in the stomach and intestine. It also relieves symptoms of periodic constipation and other digestive disorders.

A decoction made from betony has a calmative effect on the central nervous system. It is prescribed for nervous exhaustion, migraine headaches, and nervous excitability. A decoction made from the above-ground parts is a popular remedy for bladder, kidney, and liver problems, as well as for treating rheumatoid arthritis and podagra. Perhaps betony's most unconventional use in Russia is in the form of nose drops to treat arthritis and atherosclerosis.

Habitat and collection: Betony grows throughout northern Europe, the United States, and Canada. Collect the aerial parts just before the flowers bloom in the spring.

Preparation and dosage: To prepare an infusion for treating stomach problems, add 2 cups (500 ml) of boiling water to 1 tablespoon (15 g) of the herb. Steep for 2 hours. Strain and take $^1/_2$ cup (125 ml) 4 times a day 30 minutes before meals.

To make a decoction, boil 2 tablespoons (30 g) of herb for 5 minutes in 1 cup (250 ml) of water. Steep for 20 minutes. Strain and add 2 tablespoons (30 ml) of port wine. Take $^1/_3$ cup (83 ml) 3 times a day before meals.

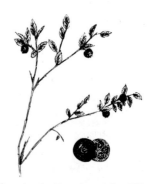

BILBERRY
Botanical name: *Vaccinium myrtillus.*
Family: Vacciniaceae.
Also known as: Huckleberry, whortleberry.

The tasty bilberry is one of the most popular berries in Russia, and millions of people venture into the forest every summer to pick them. On Sunday evenings, trains return from the country with city residents carrying buckets of bilberries they collected over the weekend. They usually cook the berries and use them as preserves during the fall and winter. In addition to tasting delicious, bilberries contain a number of important vitamins and minerals, including vitamins A and C, thiamin, chromium, iron, and copper. Bilberries also contain alkaloids, phenols, bioflavinoids, carbonic acid, and anthocyamins, which testify to the plant's numerous medicinal applications.

Parts used: Leaves, fruits.

Actions: Anodyne, antidiarrheal, astringent, disinfectant, diuretic, hemostatic, stomachic, styptic, vermicide, vulnerary.

Medicinal virtues: Russian herbalists traditionally prescribe an infusion of bilberry leaves to treat disorders of the stomach and intestinal tract, including low acidity, inflammation, and diarrhea. It is also prescribed for inflammation of the calyces of the kidneys, the mucous layer of the urinary bladder, and the liver. Bilberry infusions are also used to reduce high blood sugar. When used as a vaginal douche, a bilberry leaf infusion can relieve symptoms of leukorrhea. Cold compresses of a leaf infusion are applied to purulent skin ulcers, wounds, and eczema. It can also be given as an enema to treat hemorrhoidal bleeding.

Bilberry fruits can be used fresh, dried, or boiled. They are recommended for treating diarrhea, dysentery, and inflammation of the mucous layer of the stomach and small intestine. Herbalists also recommend bilberries to treat heartburn and as a general anti-itch remedy.

A decoction of the berries can be used to improve night vision and expel intestinal worms. It can also be taken as a gargle to relieve symptoms of tonsillitis.

Habitat and collection: Bilberry is a shrub that grows in mountainous areas of Europe, Siberia, and the northern United States. Harvest the berries during the summer when ripe. The summer is the best time to collect the leaves as well.

Preparation and dosage: To make a leaf infusion, add 1 cup (250 ml) of boiling water to 2 teaspoons (10 g) of leaves. Steep for 10 minutes and strain. Take ½ cup (125 ml) twice daily.

To prepare a fruit infusion, add 2 tablespoons (30 g) of berries to 2 cups (500 ml) of boiling hot water. Cover and let stand for 4 to 5 hours. There is no need to strain. Reheat and take warm. The suggested dosage is 1 cup (250 ml) 4 to 5 times a day before meals.

To prepare a fruit decoction, add 1 tablespoon (15 g) of dried berries to 2 cups (500 ml) of boiling water. Continue to boil gently until half the liquid evaporates. Strain. Take warm ¼ cup (62 ml) 4 times daily. This decoction is especially good for people who want to improve night vision or to expel intestinal worms. It can also be used as a gargle for tonsillitis.

To make a leaf decoction to relieve the chronic thirst of diabetics, add 1 tablespoon (15 g) of leaves to 1 cup (250 ml) of hot water. Heat to a boil, then reduce heat and simmer for 15 minutes. Filter. Take 3 to 6 cups (750 ml to 1½ liters) during the day and continue for several days until symptoms stop. If thirst returns (usually after a few weeks or months), use again for a few days.

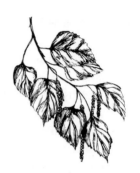

WHITE BIRCH

Botanical name: *Betula alba.*
Family: Betulaceae.
Also known as: Common birch, paper birch,
  silver birch.

The white birch tree is a plant Russian emigrés often speak about when they feel nostalgic for their homeland. The Russian term "gracious as a birch" is often used to describe a beautiful young woman, and the birch tree has long been a favorite theme of Russian poets since early czarist times.

The white birch is also widely respected for its numerous medicinal properties by both folk herbalists and official doctors. Although recognized by folk healers since the Middle Ages, written documentation concerning its medicinal properties was not published until 1834, when an article describing the use of birch leaf preparations to treat pompholyx (an acute inflammatory condition characterized by blisters on the hands and feet) appeared in *The Russian Medicine Newspaper.* The diuretic properties of birch leaves were first documented in 1894 by Russian scientists who found that birch leaf infusions could reduce edema caused by poor circulation.

Bundles of young birch branches are still widely used in traditional Russian baths (banyas) for both massage and aromatherapy. Like North Americans who tap maple trees to make maple syrup, Russians often collect the sap from birch trees in the early spring. They use the sap to make a healthful tonic that is best consumed when fresh.

Parts used: Bark, buds, leaves, sap, tar.

Actions: Analgesic, aromatic, astringent, diaphoretic, disinfectant, diuretic, tonic.

Medicinal virtues: Infusions of fresh birch leaves make an excellent natural remedy for a variety of inflammatory problems related to the bladder and kidneys. They are also believed to help prevent the formation of kidney stones. Many Russian doctors consider these infusions a more powerful medicine than those developed by the pharmaceutical industry. Birch leaf infusions also provide an additional disinfecting action that is said to relieve urinary acid diathesis. They are recommended for their ability to stimulate the flow of liver bile, which is used to digest fats. An infusion of birch buds provides an even stronger diuretic action than an infusion made from leaves.

When applied to rheumatic or arthritic joints, compresses made from mashed and steamed fresh birch leaves relieve pain and reduce inflammation.

For centuries, Russian herbalists have been using a tincture made from white birch buds to help heal wounds. They also have traditionally used a birch bud tincture as a wash to remove skin spots.

Birch sap strengthens the immune system and enhances the body's ability to resist disease. It is also considered a general tonic for the system. Birch sap is also a good diuretic and is said to reduce podagra pains. Like the tincture, birch sap applied externally helps promote wound healing. Many herbalists recommend birch sap as a wash to improve skin texture, as well as to help relieve skin problems, such as eczema and pimples. It is also used on the scalp to remove dandruff and increase hair growth.

Birch tar is good for treating skin diseases and promotes wound healing. It is even a primary ingredient in a number of commercially prepared ointments available in Russian pharmacies with a doctor's prescription.

Habitat and collection: The white birch grows in woodlands throughout Europe, northern Asia, and in North America, from Labrador south to Pennsylvania and west to Montana and Alaska. Harvest the buds in late March or April and the leaves during the late spring or early summer. When harvesting the bark, do not take off bark around the entire circumference of the trunk, or the tree will die.

Collect the sap during the winter. Make a diagonal cut from 3 to 6 inches long in the trunk of a tree that is at least several years old. Insert a thin (1/4-inch-thick) peeled branch into the lower end of the cut and aim it downward. The sap will drip along the branch. Place a container under the branch, and collect the sap for 1 or 2 days. Make sure that the container is covered to prevent leaves and other matter from falling in. Filter the sap.

Preparation and dosage: To make an infusion, add 1 cup (250 ml) of boiling water to 1 or 2 tablespoons (15 to 30 g) of fresh leaves or buds. Allow to steep for 10 minutes. Drink 1 cup (250 ml) 3 times a day after meals.

To make a tonic, filter the sap, which will have a watery consistency. It can be kept under refrigeration for up to 1 week. Drink 3 to 4 cups daily for up to several months.

BISTORT

Botanical name: *Polygonum bistorta.*
Family: Polygonaceae.
Also known as: Dragonwort, patience dock,
  red legs, sweet dock.

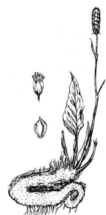

Bistort grows in meadows and near streams in the Caucasus and Ural mountains as well as in other parts of northern Europe. Russians call this hearty plant "serpentine" because of the serpentlike shape of its root. It is also called "crawfish's neck" because the root is somewhat flat on two sides and appears to be pleated in form.

Bistort has long been used as a food in Europe. The plant itself is rich in starch, and is a natural astringent as well. Eating bistort in times of famine was said to shrink the intestines, thus reducing the amount of food needed to relieve hunger. Bistort root was also an ingredient in an astringent tonic wine, which was used to treat people suffering from general debility and tuberculosis. The roasted roots of an American relative of this plant *(Polygonum bistortoides)* were enjoyed by the Cheyenne and Blackfoot, who ate them alone or mixed into stews.

Parts used: Rootstocks.

Actions: Antibacterial, anti-inflammatory, astringent, diuretic.

Medicinal virtues: Since the roots of the plant contain 15 to 25 percent tannin, it is used as an astringent mouthwash for inflammations of the mouth and gums, including stomatitis, gingivitis, and periodontitis. Taken internally, bistort is an excellent remedy for treating diarrhea and dysentery, although extended use can cause constipation. It is also used as a gargle to help relieve symptoms of tonsillitis.

Because of its astringent and antibacterial properties, Russian herbalists in centuries past recommended bistort to treat venereal diseases like gonorrhea. It is used as both a wash and a poultice to treat skin sores and to control bleeding. When applied directly to a wound, the powdered roots will stop bleeding.

Habitat and collection: Bistort grows in damp soil in meadows and near streams. Harvest only the rootstock.

Preparation and dosage: To prepare a decoction, add 1 teaspoon (5 g) of rootstock to 1 cup (250 ml) of water. Boil for 20 minutes. Strain. Take 1 tablespoon (15 ml) 30 minutes before meals 2 to 3 times a day. It can also be used as a mouthwash or gargle at this dosage.

———

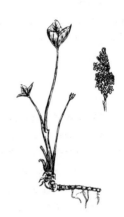

BUCKBEAN

Botanical name: *Menyanthes trifoliata.*
Family: Menyanthaceae.
Also known as: Bogbean, bean trefoil, marsh trefoil.

The Russian name for this herb, *vahta*, comes from an old folk legend about a girl of that name. When Vahta was little, she would play in the forest with gnomes and listen to their stories about herbs and other plants. But one day her spiteful stepmother, who was a witch, turned her into a mermaid and banished her to life at the bottom of a river.

Vahta spent many lonely months living in the river, but one day she left to play with her forest friends once more. She forgot that she had to return to the river by sundown, and when she finally returned late in the evening, the Queen of the Underwater Kingdom punished her severely. She made Vahta stand guard at the entrances of all rivers and lakes, never to venture into the forest again. Since that time local people began to notice a plant with a beautiful white and rose flower that looked like a weeping mermaid. The flowers were so brilliant they could be seen even at night and were always a sign that a river, lake, or swamp was nearby.

Parts used: Leaves

Actions: Antiphlogistic, cholagogue, digestive, febrifuge, laxative, tonic.

Medicinal virtues: Russian medical science foresees that buckbean, presently prescribed for a wide variety of diseases, will be used even more in the future. Throughout the former Soviet Union, buckbean is used to treat gastritis (with low acidity), intestinal colic, constipation, and meteorism, a distention by gas in the abdomen or intestines. For these health problems, a cold extract is usually prescribed.

Russian folk medicine has long considered buckbean to be a very good bitter tonic to increase the appetite before meals. A decoction is often prescribed for patients suffering from tuberculosis, colds, and coughs, as well as for diseases of the liver.

Preparations of buckbean are used externally as an antiseptic to wash fresh wounds as well as older wounds that are slow to heal. It is also used for skin ulcers and other skin diseases.

Habitat and collection: Buckbean grows in bogs, marshes, and shallow water in northern Europe and North America. Harvest the leaves during the summer.

Preparation and dosage: To make an infusion add 1¼ cups (300 ml) of hot water to 2 tablespoons (30 g) of dried leaves. Steep for 15 minutes, then cool for 45 minutes. Filter and press the last drops of liquid from the leaves. Take ⅓ cup (80 ml) 3 times a day a half hour before meals.

To prepare a cold extract, put 1 tablespoon (15 g) of dried leaves in 1 cup (250 ml) of cold water. Let stand for 8 hours and filter. Drink ½ cup (125 ml) twice a day before meals.

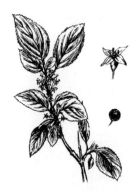

BUCKTHORN
Botanical name: *Rhamnus cathartica.*
Family: Rhamnaceae.
Also known as: Ramsthorn.

Buckthorn has been known to European herbalists for at least a thousand years and was included in Anglo-Saxon herbals before the Norman conquest. There was even a superstition that Christ's crown of thorns was made of buckthorn.

This herb was first introduced to the Russian medical community during the eighteenth century. Botanists were sent by the Imperial Academy of Science in St. Petersburg to small communities and farms all over Russia to collect and classify herbs. The botanists would also interview local herbalists and farmers to find out how the herbs were used. The herbs were brought back to St. Petersburg for more extensive study in the laboratory. They were classified according to their Latin families, species, and genera.

As a result, Russian botanists were able to assemble detailed scientific reports that could be understood by botanists and other researchers throughout Europe.

During one of these expeditions, the botanists found that buckthorn had been used by folk herbalists to treat a wide variety of digestive problems for centuries. Even to this day, buckthorn preparations are used by folk and official herbalists alike, and commercial buckthorn extract is available in Russian pharmacies.

Parts used: Bark, branches, fruit.

Actions: Analgesic, anti-inflammatory, purgative.

Medicinal virtues: A decoction or infusion made from the fruits of this herb is a very effective remedy for chronic constipation, hemorrhoids, and anal irritation. In folk medicine, a decoction made from branches is used to treat stomach ulcers. Externally, it is used as a compress for cuts. A decoction made from buckthorn bark is recommended to treat gastritis due to hyperacidity.

Habitat and collection: Buckthorn is often a common hedge plant and is found in Europe, Asia, the northeastern United States, and southeastern Canada. Collect the berries in September and October. Before collecting them, study an illustration of the plant carefully. Make sure that the berries you pick are buckthorn. Other plants growing nearby may also have black berries that could be poisonous. After collection, dry the berries in sunlight for the first day or two. Continue the drying process in a warm (but not hot) oven.

Preparation and dosage: To make a decoction, add 2 teaspoons (10 g) of dried crushed fruit to 1 cup (250 ml) of boiling water. Simmer for 15 to 30 minutes. Strain. Take 1 tablespoon (15 ml) 3 to 4 times a day. A course of treatment should not exceed two weeks.

Buckthorn reduces fermentation in the stomach and intestines and acts as an anti-inflammative and analgesic. Herbalists recommend that people suffering from stomach and intestinal distress chew several fresh buckthorn berries in the morning on an empty stomach.

Caution: Several fruits should cause no unpleasant side effects, but too high a dose can induce diarrhea and vomiting in sensitive people. At the first sign of adverse symptoms, the course of treatment should be stopped unless a qualified health-care professional recommends otherwise.

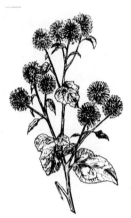

BURDOCK
Botanical name: *Arctium lappa.*
Family: Compositae.
Also known as: Burr seed, cockleburr.

Burdock is a very old herb in Russia. Historical evidence shows that burdock was used by the physician of Prince Alexander Nevsky, the famous Russian military leader who defeated the German crusaders in 1240.

It is difficult to explain why this herb is called *lopuh* in Russian. Referring to someone as a *lopuh* is like calling a person a fool in English: someone who constantly lets himself be deceived by others. Perhaps this term is used because of the greenish gray fruits of the burdock. These small prickly balls catch on the clothing and skin of anyone (whether human or beast) who touches the plant while walking through the meadow. When people pull the burdock fruits off their clothes, they unwittingly enable the plant to propagate in a new location.

Parts used: Leaves, roots, seeds (fruits).

Actions: Anodyne, antiseptic, aperient, cholagogue, diaphoretic, diuretic, emollient.

Medicinal virtues: Preparations of burdock are used to treat podagra, inflammatory diseases of the kidneys, gall and kidney stones, gastritis, colic, hemorrhoids, and diabetes. In traditional Russian herbal medicine, burdock is used for treating a wide variety of skin diseases, including itchiness, eczema, rashes, and boils. It is taken both internally and externally. An oil extract of the roots is applied to the scalp to prevent baldness. A combination of bruised or pounded leaves and an oil extract of the roots are recommended for wounds. Burdock is considered most effective when taken in an infusion containing bilberry leaves and green beans.

Habitat and collection: Burdock is found throughout northern Europe and North America, mainly on roadsides and in meadows and damp places. It is often cultivated in gardens. The roots and leaves are usually collected in July, while the flowers can be harvested whenever they are in bloom.

Preparation and dosage: In 1968 the Russian physician A. P. Popov introduced an original method for treating eczema with preparations of burdock. He recommends placing 4 ounces (100 grams) of dried, powdered roots in a 5-quart (5-liter) enamel pot and filling the pot with boiling water. Continue to boil for 20 minutes and let cool to 102 to 104°F (39 to 40°C). Next, take a cotton sheet, fold it lengthwise into four quarters, and moisten it well with the extract, carefully squeezing out excess moisture. Wrap the nude patient from the armpits to the ankles in the sheet. Wrap the patient in another dry sheet and have him or her lie down (and preferably sleep) for 1 to 2 hours. The best time to do this is before bedtime. You can repeat these body wraps for up to 6 days. The eczema should begin to heal within 1 to 2 days.

To make an infusion, add 1 cup (250 ml) of boiling water to 2 tablespoons (30 g) of leaves. Steep for 2 hours. Filter. Drink ½ cup (125 ml) (warm) 2 to 4 times a day after eating.

To make a decoction, put 2 tablespoons (30 g) of dried roots in 1 cup (250 ml) of cold water. Simmer over low heat for 30 minutes, stirring often. Let cool for 10 minutes and filter. Take ½ cup (125 ml) 2 or 3 times a day after eating; heat before drinking. Store in a cool, dark place for a maximum of 3 days.

To make an oil extract, put 4 tablespoons (60 g) of dried, powdered roots in 3½ ounces (100 ml) of vegetable oil. Cook over low heat for 15 minutes, stirring occasionally. For external use.

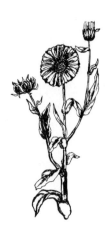

CALENDULA

Botanical name: *Calendula officinalis*
Family: Compositae.
Also known as: Marigold, holigold, Mary bud.

This herb has been used for centuries in Russian folk medicine. The medicinal use of this herb can probably be traced to ancient Greece. The Greek physician Diascorides, who used calendula to treat gallstones and diseases of the liver, is the first to mention using the herb medicinally.

Russians developed their own traditions over the years, and calendula was eventually cultivated especially for pharmaceutical use. At the present time, entire farms are devoted to the cultivation of this valuable herb. Over the past thirty years a number of scientific studies have been carried out to discover the chemical and biological properties of this herb, including its possible value as an anticancer remedy. The All-Union Institute of Herbs developed a new variety of calendula (known as *rejick*) especially for use in official Russian medicine.

Parts used: Flowers, leaves.

Actions: Antibacterial, antifungal, antiphlogistic, antiseptic, emollient, sedative, tonic, vulnerary.

Medicinal virtues: Calendula has a wide range of medicinal effects. As mentioned before, preparations of this herb have long been used to treat diseases of the liver and to break up gallstones. It has also been used to treat stomach spasms and indigestion. In 1988 a number of Russian studies revealed that preparations of calendula have a tonic effect on the heart and can help normalize heart activity. At the same time, it can reduce blood pressure and edema. Russian women use calendula both to delay menstruation and to help relieve the severity of painful periods.

Antibacterial and anti-inflammatory, calendula is effective for treating tonsillitis and diseases of the mucous membrane of the mouth. It is also used for treating internal and external fungal infections. Calendula ointment (known as *Unguentum calendula*), readily available in Russian pharmacies, is applied to cuts, wounds, and burns.

Habitat and collection: A popular garden plant, calendula flowers can be harvested from June to October.

Preparation and dosage: To make an infusion, add 1 cup (250 ml) of boiling water to 1 tablespoon (15 g) of dried flowers. Steep for 10 minutes. Strain. Take 1 tablespoon (15 ml) 3 to 5 times a day.

To make a decoction, pour 2 cups (500 ml) of water into a pot containing 1 tablespoon (15 g) of dried flowers. Boil for 5 minutes. Allow to stand for 45 minutes at room temperature. Strain. Take 1 tablespoon (15 ml) 3 to 4 times a day.

To prepare a tincture, soak a handful of dried flowers in 2 cups (500 ml) of whisky. Allow to stand for 4 weeks. Take 5 to 20 drops daily as needed.

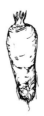

CARROT (WILD)
Botanical name: *Daucus carota.*
Family: Umbelliferae.
Also known as: Queen Anne's lace, bird's nest.

The wild carrot has been known in Russia since prehistoric times and has been an important herb and staple food for tens of thousands of years. The wild carrot, which once grew throughout Russia and Europe, was not orange like the carrot that is widely cultivated today but had a tough, whitish, inedible root. The carrot as we know it today was developed in the seventeenth century.

Known primarily as Queen Anne's lace, wild carrot is the subject of a myth concerning its appearance. One early story says that a queen named Anne was making lace when she pricked her finger on a needle. The purple floret at the center of the flower represents a drop of blood which fell onto the lace from her finger. However, others believe that the flower is not named after Queen Anne, but Saint Anne, the mother of the Virgin Mary. It happens that Saint Anne is the patron saint of lacemakers. Since the flower indeed appears to feature delicate lacework, it is named after her.

Parts used: Leaves, roots, seeds.

Actions: Antilithic, carminative, diuretic, stimulant.

Medicinal virtues: Wild carrot infusions have long been used in Russia to treat chronic kidney diseases and diseases of the bladder, including kidney stones. They are also helpful in relieving urinary disorders, including cystitis and prostatitis. An infusion of seeds and roots is used to increase the flow of urine. In Russia, the boiled mashed root of the wild carrot is often prescribed as a poultice to treat burns, wounds, and cuts. One-half teaspoon of bruised or crushed wild carrot seeds, eaten directly, is considered effective in reducing flatulence and expelling intestinal worms.

Habitat and collection: Native to eastern Europe and western Asia, but widely naturalized in North America, the wild carrot is found in open fields and waste places and by the roadside. Harvest the mature seeds and leaves in late summer. The roots can be collected in the fall.

Preparation and dosage: To make an infusion, put 1 teaspoon (5 g) of the dried seeds in 1 cup (250 ml) of hot water. Steep for 10 to 15 minutes. Strain. Take ⅓ cup (80 ml) 3 times daily.

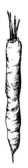

CARROT (CULTIVATED)
Botanical name: *Daucus carota.*
Family: Umbelliferae.

The carrot as we know it today is a subspecies *(sativa)* of wild carrot *(Daucus carota)*, which was just described. The first domestic carrots were cultivated in Europe five hundred years ago and were mostly purple in color. Over the years, yellow varieties were developed, followed by the familiar orange varieties we eat today. The domestic carrot was first introduced to North America by settlers to the Jamestown Colony in Virginia in the 1600s. The seeds were soon shared with local Native Americans, who began growing carrots themselves.

Parts used: Roots.

Actions: Anthelmintic, antispasmodic, cardiac, carminative, diuretic, galactagogue, hepatic, laxative, stimulant, stomachic.

Medicinal virtues: The juice of the cultivated carrot is considered a universal remedy to treat vitamin deficiency and especially anemia. It reduces chronic fatigue and increases the appetite. Russian herbalists prescribe carrot juice with honey or grated carrots in milk to increase resistance to colds.

Fresh carrot juice is also recommended for skin lesions and for problems of the gastrointestinal tract. It has a favorable effect on the pancreatic function and improves the exchange functions of the liver and kidneys. It is used in Russia to treat chronic or acute cholecystitis and for different forms of cholelithiasis and urolithiasis. The juice is also recommended for treating cardiovascular problems, especially cardiac insufficiency and stenocardia. A carrot juice gargle is reputed to heal throat infections.

Carrot promotes the production of milk in nursing mothers. Like garlic, it is an antimicrobial and anthelmintic and can be used to destroy threadworm and seatworm in the intestinal tract. It is also well known for improving vision, especially at night.

A salad made from carrots, cranberries, and cabbage is rich in iodine and is recommended by Russian herbalists as part of a weight-loss program. Carrot eaten alone is said to help people control diabetes. Finely grated fresh carrots (in the form of gruel) can be placed on the skin to relieve burns, cuts, and infected wounds. Grated carrot can also be eaten to relieve symptoms of constipation, and an infusion made from carrot leaves is used in Russia to reduce and eliminate hemorrhoids.

Habitat and collection: Carrots are cultivated throughout the world, preferably in light, sandy soil that is well fertilized. The roots are usually harvested in September and October.

Preparation and dosage: Drink 1 cup (250 ml) or more of fresh carrot juice daily as desired.

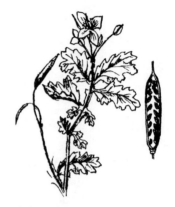

CELANDINE
Botanical name: *Chelidonium majus.*
Family: Papaveraceae.
Also known as: Greater celandine.

As with other herb names, the Russian word for celandine, *chistotel,* which means "body-cleansing," is self-explanatory. Russian folklore tells of a princess named Natasha who lived toward the end of the twelfth century. Her husband was killed by a rival prince, who was also his brother. The killer wanted to take Natasha for his wife, but both of them were suddenly stricken with a terrible skin disease, known today as eczema.

The prince, feeling guilty for having murdered his brother, threw himself into a river to cleanse his sins and died. Still covered with eczema, Natasha took to the forest, where she slept on the ground and lived with wild animals. One day God gave her a way to heal her body. As she walked through the forest, she brushed against a celandine plant, and it removed the eczema completely.

Parts used: Aerial parts.

Actions: Anodyne, anti-inflammatory, antispasmodic, caustic, cholagogue, diaphoretic, diuretic, hydragogue, purgative, vulnerary.

Medicinal virtues: Russian official medicine uses preparations from the orange latex of the stem for removing warts, freckles, corns, and fungal diseases. Dr. V. C. Yagodka, working in the Kiev State Institute for Advanced Medical Training of the Ukraine Health Ministry, found that the herb inhibits cancerous growths on the skin. He applies it to areas where cancerous skin growths have been surgically removed, and the celandine preparation prevents them from recurring.

Some of the chemical substances found in the herb can calm the nervous system, expel bile, and tone the muscles of the uterus. Celandine is also used internally to treat infections of the gallbladder and to help dissolve gallstones. However, physicians stress that this herb should be taken internally under medical supervision only.

Habitat and collection: Celandine is a hearty plant and grows in rich, damp soil in eastern Russia, northern Europe, and the northeastern United States. It can often be found growing near fences, roadsides, and hedges. The leaves and flowers are collected when they bloom, usually in May or June. They are then dried in a shady place. Roots should be unearthed in late summer and also dried in a shady place.

Preparation and dosage: To make an infusion, add 1 cup (250 ml) of boiling water to 1 teaspoon (5 g) of the herb. Allow to steep for 30 minutes. Drink ¹/₂ cup (125 ml) at room temperature daily.

To make juice, run the fresh herb and roots through a food grinder. Place the mash in cheesecloth and squeeze out the juice. Dab a small amount on affected areas of the skin no more than 3 times a day.

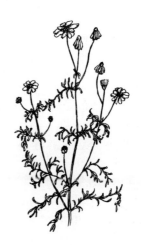

CHAMOMILE
Botanical name: *Matricaria chamomilla.*
Family: Compositae.
Also known as: Common chamomile,
   German chamomile, wild chamomile,
   Hungarian chamomile.

Chamomile grows widely throughout Russia and other former Soviet republics and is among the best-known and most appreciated native plants. It would be very difficult to find a Russian family who has not had firsthand experience with this herb.

Russians regard chamomile, with its long stem and delicate white petals surrounding a bright yellow center, as a flower of exceptional beauty. Young village girls traditionally collect the flowers and braid them together to make garlands for their hair. Another old tradition parallels the use of the daisy in North America. A young man or woman picks a chamomile flower and begins to remove each petal saying "He [she] loves me, he [she] loves me not," with the last petal declaring the truth.

From an herbalist's perspective, the chamomile is not only a beautiful flower but a powerful healing plant with a wide range of therapeutic applications.

Parts used: Flowers.

Actions: Analgesic, anodyne, antiphlogistic, antiseptic, antispasmodic, calmative, carminative, diaphoretic, stomachic, tonic.

Medicinal virtues: Chamomile is renowned throughout Russia for its relaxing, anti-inflammatory, and carminative properties. Chamomile infusions are perhaps best known for treating digestive problems, especially those involving inflammation of the stomach mucosa. It is also valued for the treatment of both acute and chronic gastritis, stomach and duodenal ulcers, and colitis. Chamomile reduces the fermentation processes in the digestive tract and increases the secretion of bile from the liver.

Research indicates that the herb stimulates the immune system's infection-fighting white blood cells. Chamomile is recommended for treating liver, gallbladder, kidney, and urinary bladder problems, as well as urethritis and gastritis. Taken at bedtime, chamomile tea promotes restful sleep and is often recommended for people with insomnia. The tea is also used to treat a variety of nervous disorders and pain caused by neuritis and neuralgia. Russian herbalists have also recommended chamomile tea for the treatment of bronchial asthma, tonsillitis, laryngitis, rheumatic problems, painful joints, lumbago, and gout. Chamomile may also help reduce the inflammation that accompanies arthritis. Chamomile infusions taken internally are valued by folk dermatologists to treat eczema, neurodermatitis, hives (nettle rash), and prurigo.

A tea made from chamomile flowers, valerian root, mint leaves, caraway, and fennel taken in equal parts relieves intestinal cramps and spasms, as well as symptoms of meteorism.

When used as a gargle or mouthwash, chamomile tea is useful for treating gingivitis, stomatitis, and tonsillitis. Russian doctors use chamomile drops to treat ear infections. Chamomile douches are also used in Russia to treat women's disorders, including menstrual cramps and uterine hemorrhage.

Used externally, chamomile infusions are recommended for treating allergic dermatitis and ulcers of the lower leg. A wash can soothe irritated eyes, as well as help relieve hemorrhoids and heal open wounds and boils. Some use a chamomile infusion as a rinse for blond hair.

Habitat and collection: Native to southern Europe, chamomile grows wild in fields. It is also cultivated extensively throughout the world. Gather the flowers from May through August.

Preparation and dosage: Chamomile infusions are very pleasant to the taste and are among the most popular herbal teas. To make an infusion, add

1 teaspoon (5 g) of dried flowers to one cup (250 ml) of boiling water. Steep for 10 minutes and strain. Add a touch of honey if you wish. Drink 1 cup (250 ml) 3 times a day after meals to relieve digestive problems, or 1 cup (250 ml) at bedtime to facilitate restful sleep.

To make a chamomile rinse, add 1 tablespoon (15 g) of dried flowers to 1 quart (1 liter) of hot water. Steep for 15 minutes, strain, and allow to cool to room temperature.

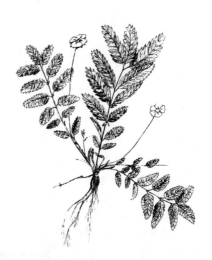

CINQUEFOIL
Botanical name: *Potentilla anserina.*
Family: Rosaceae.
Also known as: Five-finger grass,
    five-leaf grass.

The Russian name for this herb means "like goose feet," because the shape of this herb is reminiscent of goose feet. Early Russians found this herb growing wild everywhere and originally used it as a source of food. They used young fresh leaves in salads and soups and boiled and ate the root. Mashed leaves were considered a good addition to various fish and meat dishes. While not known primarily as a major food source today, gourmet vegetarian chefs might consider the many uses of the cinquefoil plant. As an early Russian food and as an exotic new plant to add to modern menus, the humble cinquefoil has no unpleasant side effects.

Parts used: Aerial parts.

Actions: Anodyne, antispasmodic, astringent, diuretic, emmenagogue, hemostatic, laxative, vulnerary.

Medicinal virtues: An infusion of cinquefoil can relieve spasms of the smooth muscles of the gastrointestinal tract. It is recommended for catarrh of the stomach and intestines, as well as for stomach ulcers, constipation, diarrhea, and dysentery. Russian folk healers use the herbal infusion (made with goat milk) as a diuretic. Infusions are good for kidney, bladder, and liver disorders. Infusions also help regulate the body's metabolism for people suffering from diabetes, goiter, and obesity.

A cinquefoil infusion in water is recommended for relieving menstrual cramps, toothache, and bleeding gums. As an astringent, a gargle is helpful for treating mouth sores, and an external wash is often used for relief of dermatitis and skin rash.

In folk medicine, a cinquefoil decoction is valued for treating stomach problems. Cinquefoil powder is added to fried eggs for a unique treatment for dysentery. A decoction of this herb is also used to treat uterine hemorrhage and excessive menstrual flow, as well as for nervous cramps and spasms in children.

Cinquefoil juice may be taken internally for chronic gallbladder inflammation or applied externally for healing wounds, eczema, and hemorrhoids.

Habitat and collection: Cinquefoil grows wild in fields and marshes in Europe and North America. Harvest from May through September.

Preparation and dosage: To make an infusion, add 2 teaspoons (10 g) of the herb to 1 cup (250 ml) of hot water. Allow to steep for 15 minutes. Take 1/2 cup (125 ml) 4 to 5 times a day before meals. For external use, add 1 tablespoon (15 g) of herb to 2 cups (500 ml) of water. Cover and allow to stand for two hours. Then bring to a boil, remove from the flame, and let stand for an additional two hours.

To prepare a decoction for internal use, add 2 teaspoons (10 g) of dried, powdered herb to 1 cup (250 ml) of boiling water. Boil for 20 minutes. Strain. Take 1 tablespoon (15 ml) 6 to 8 times throughout the day.

To prepare a juice for interal or external use, use fresh aerial parts and follow directions given in "Making Herbal Preparations." Take 1/3 cup 4 times a day. This juice can also be used to clean wounds.

CLINKER POLYPORE

Botanical name: *Inonotus obligus* [Fr.] pil.,
  also *Poria obliqua.*
Family: Poloyporaceae.
Also known as: Birch canker polypore.

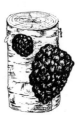

This is one Russian medicinal that is not found in other herbal traditions. *Inonotus obligus* is a fungus (known in Old Russia as *chaga*) that grows on birch trees in many parts of the country. Although for centuries traditional Russian healers or knowledgists have considered it one of the most powerful medicinal elements, chaga was not studied officially by Soviet medical science until the second half of the twentieth century. At the present time, several institutes are conducting ongoing research, so the information we offer here is based primarily on previous discoveries by both the knowledgists and official Soviet medicine.

The fungus is approximately 10 to 16 inches (25 to 40 cm) in size and deeply cracked. Chaga is black, with the fertile portion dark brown. Its spores are broadly elliptical, smooth, and white to light yellow.

Parts used: Fungus.

Actions: Antiemetic, aperient, cathartic, tonic.

Medicinal virtues: Preparations made from chaga are believed to reduce the growth of both benign and malignant growths and help normalize activity in the intestinal tract. The chaga extract is used to help reduce the size of cancerous growths when surgery and radiation are not deemed advisable. It has been used during chemotherapy for cancer patients, although a special diet based primarily on vegetables and dairy products is often recommended to accompany the use of chaga. A commercial extract of chaga, known in the Soviet Union as *befungin,* contains one-half chaga extract, chlorine, and sulfur of cobalt and is used to treat patients suffering from cancer.

Chaga alleviates diseases of the stomach and the intestinal tract, especially if these problems are accompanied by a decrease of excretions. Chaga also reduces vomiting and abdominal pain while it helps normalize the activity of the intestinal tract.

Habitat and collection: This fungus grows in black birch trees in the forests of Russia, western Europe, Canada, and the northeastern United States. Chaga can be collected throughout the year, but traditional Russian herbalists prefer autumn and spring. It is important to distinguish true chaga from false chaga (which does not possess the same powerful healing properties and should not be taken internally) by the underside of the fungus. True chaga can be identified by its serrated edge on the undersurface, while false chaga is smooth.

Do not harvest chaga from dead or dying trees or use fungus that is completely black in color (i.e., penetrating throughout its thickness) or otherwise past its prime. Chaga is very hard, so it is usually removed from the tree with a sharp ax.

After harvesting, the fungus is cut into $1^1/_4$- to $2^1/_2$-inch (3- to 6-cm) pieces and dried in a well-ventilated dark room. It can also be laid out on a pan and dried in an oven set at 140°F (60°C). As it dries, the fungus will become more solid and firm and will take on a dark brown color. It should be stored in a glass jar for a maximum of 2 years.

Preparation and dosage: Here is a traditional Russian preparation for chaga extract:

1. Pour 2.5 quarts (2.5 liters) of boiling water over 2 cups (500 ml) of dry chaga. Cover and let stand at room temperature for 4 days.
2. Filter and refrigerate the liquid in a covered container. Reserve chaga.
3. Grind the chaga in a food grinder or processor to a mushy consistency.
4. Add 2 quarts (2 liters) of water at 122°F (50°C) to the ground chaga, and let stand at room temperature for 48 hours.
5. Strain mixture through a cheesecloth filter and squeeze the chaga until it is dry. Discard chaga.
6. Add the liquid from step 1 to the liquid from step 4. Cover and refrigerate.

You should now have approximately 3 quarts (3 liters) of the chaga preparation, which should last for 4 days. (After 4 days it is no longer any good.) Drink $^3/_4$ cup (200 ml) 4 times a day before meals.

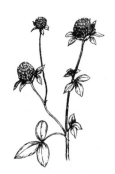

RED CLOVER

Botanical name: *Trifolium pratense.*
Family: Papilonaceae.
Also known as: Wild clover.

Nature generously distributed red clover, a modest and unremarkable plant, in fields and meadows, and humans discovered a multitude of ways to use it for their benefit. If we could imagine our earliest years as a species, we would find that our ancestors observed other animals consuming these plants as an essential food and tried to see how they could be useful to humans as well. Their experiences were collected over hundreds of generations, giving red clover a prominent place in traditional folk medicine. Today, Russian scientists have researched red clover extensively with contemporary methods and have awarded this humble herb a prominent place in Russian official medicine.

Russians have long used red clover in daily life as a dye to color fabrics and as a baking additive to improve the quality of bread. It is also a popular caffeine-free tea. Yet Russian herbalists have also recognized red clover for its ability to treat a variety of diseases.

Parts used: Flowers with top leaves, roots.

Actions: Alterative, anodyne, antispasmodic, cholagogue, diaphoretic, diuretic, expectorant, hemostatic, tonic, vulnerary.

Medicinal virtues: Taken internally, an infusion of red clover is recommended for treating colds (and coughs due to colds), as well as bronchitis and bronchial asthma. In Russian folk medicine, red clover infusions are also used to treat anemia, emaciation, asthenia, and diabetes mellitus. They also promote the onset of menstruation, relieve cramps and spasms, and treat uterine hemorrhage (metrorrhagia). Folk dermatologists recommend drinking red clover infusions to treat allergic skin conditions including vitiligo, vasculitis, childhood eczema, and balding. Red clover infusions are also used externally to relieve inflammation of the ears and eyes.

A decoction made of leaves and flowers is prescribed to treat a wide variety of health complaints, including chest pain, malaria, chronic rheumatism, kidney problems, and inflammation of the bladder. As a tonic, a red clover decoction makes an effective stomach remedy. A decoction made from roots is a traditional folk remedy to relieve inflammation of the ovaries and to reduce the size of benign fibroid tumors.

In Russia, red clover tincture is recommended to help reduce serum cholesterol and is considered an effective preventive for atherosclerosis. It is also used as part of a complex remedy for treating tuberculosis.

Traditional Russian herbalists recommend taking red clover juice internally to treat symptoms of jaundice. Mothers bathe their children in baths containing red clover juice to heal rickets. In addition, poultices made from red clover leaves are placed on wounds, burns, scalds, swellings, and furuncles and are recommended for treating dermatitis and hypercelatosis. Red clover juice, when rubbed into the roots of graying hair, is reputed to make it revert to its original color.

Habitat and collection: Red clover is found in fields and meadows throughout Europe and North America. Gather the flowers and leaves from May through September.

Preparation and dosage: To prepare an infusion, add 1 to 2 tablespoons (15 to 30 g) of leaves and flowers to 1 cup (250 ml) of hot water. Allow to steep for 10 minutes and strain. Take 1 cup (250 ml), drinking slowly.

To make a decoction, steep 2 teaspoons (10 g) of roots in a cup of water for 30 minutes. Strain and press out any excess liquid. Add enough water to make 1 cup (250 ml) of liquid. Take 1 tablespoon (15 g) 4 to 5 times a day before meals.

To use a tincture, take 5 to 30 drops of root decoction 3 times a day in 1 cup (250 ml) of water.

To make a juice for external application, use fresh leaves, flowers, stems, and/or roots and process according to directions given in "Making Herbal Preparations." It is not necessary to heat red clover juice unless it will be stored for more than 2 or 3 days.

COLTSFOOT

Botanical name: *Tussilago farfara.*
Family: Compositae.
Also known as: Bullsfoot, coughwort,
  horsehoof.

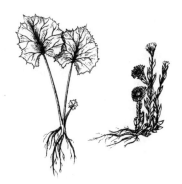

Russians call this herb "mother and stepmother" because of the unusual structure of the leaves. The underside of the leaves is soft while the upper side is hard, like the stereotypical stepmother of Russian folklore.

Parts used: Flowers, leaves.

Actions: Antiphlogistic, astringent, demulcent, emollient, expectorant.

Medicinal virtues: In Russia official medical practitioners use coltsfoot both alone and with other herbs as a tea to treat diseases of the mouth, throat, larynx, and bronchial tubes, such as coughs, colds, hoarseness, bronchitis, bronchial asthma, pleurisy, and throat catarrh. It is also prescribed for diseases of the kidneys, catarrh of the urinary bladder, and for headache. Coltsfoot is also sometimes used to treat diarrhea.

Russian folk healers have traditionally used coltsfoot externally to treat boils, chronic skin ulcers, insect bites, burns, and phlebitis. Pounded leaves are dried and smoked like tobacco to relieve shortness of breath and headache.

Habitat and collection: Coltsfoot favors loamy and limestone soils and is found in Russia, much of western Europe, and the United States. It can usually be found in waste areas, pastures, and meadows, as well as on railroad and highway embankments. Harvest the flowers as soon as they are open.

Preparation and dosage: To prepare an infusion, steep 1 tablespoon (15 g) of leaves or flowers in 1 cup (250 ml) of hot water for 30 minutes. Strain. Sweeten with honey (if desired) and consume ¹/₃ to ¹/₂ cup (80 to 125 ml) twice a day 1 hour before eating. The infusion should be taken warm.

To make a decoction, add 1 teaspoon (5 g) of leaves to 2 cups (500 ml) of boiling water. Continue to boil for another 5 to 7 minutes. Take ¹/₃ to ¹/₂ cup (80 to 125 ml) 2 or 3 times daily 1 hour before meals.

Coltsfoot juice can be taken internally or applied to the skin. Prepare according to directions given in "Making Herbal Preparations." Take

1 tablespoon (15 ml) of juice 3 times daily an hour before meals. Apply fresh crushed leaves directly to the skin to treat skin problems and phlebitis.

Caution: **Coltsfoot contains pyrrolizidine alkaloid senkirkine, a potentially toxic chemical that affects the liver. Most herbalists consider coltsfoot to be safe when taken at the recommended doses for a maximum of 4 weeks. No more than 2 courses of treatment are recommended per year.**

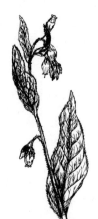

COMFREY
Botanical name: *Symphytum officinale.*
Family: Boraginaceae.
Also known as: Knitbone, knitback,
   healing herb, ass ear.

Russian soldiers have used comfrey as a handy field remedy since czarist times. Handwritten journals describe cavalry soldiers who "sliced and slew comfrey roots to mash" and applied them to each other's wounds, holding them on "until the blood stopped and the groans of pain were gone." During those times, comfrey was known as "knit-together herb."

But the weapons of battle changed and the name of the herb changed as well. The widespread use of cannons and guns forced soldiers to fight from trenches, and they actually dug up comfrey from the edge of the trench. Although comfrey was no longer needed to treat injuries caused by sabres and swords, its antibacterial and styptic properties made it a popular remedy for treating bullet and shrapnel wounds. Modern Russian herbalists soon adopted the name "trench herb."

Parts used: Roots, sometimes fresh leaves.

Actions: Antibacterial, antidiarrheal, antiphlogistic, expectorant, hemostatic, laxative, mucilaginous, stomachic, styptic, vulnerary.

Medicinal virtues: Although Russian official medicine is still conducting research on comfrey and warns against taking it in large doses internally, Russian folk healers use comfrey extensively. As official research continues, many folk healers believe that comfrey preparations will become an authorized herb for Russian physicians to prescribe for their patients.

Traditional folk healers have long used comfrey root preparations to speed the healing of wounds. They have also used it extensively to promote the mending of broken bones and reduce inflammation around the site of the break.

Folk herbalists have also found that comfrey preparations reduce pain of the intestinal tract, improve digestive processes, and heal damaged mucous membranes of the stomach and intestines. They also prescribe comfrey decoctions for treating chronic inflammation of the stomach and intestines, as well as to relieve symptoms of dysentery, gastritis, and stomach ulcers. Because comfrey is an excellent expectorant, folk herbalists also prescribe comfrey decoctions for tuberculosis and chronic bronchitis.

In *Herbs of Siberia Used for Cardiovascular Diseases,* Dr. I. M. Krasnoborov and Dr. S. B. Kaznacheev report that comfrey can reduce blood pressure and facilitate breathing. Although some physicians caution that large doses of comfrey taken internally can injure the central nervous system and the liver, testimonies to the value of this herb can be found in nearly all Russian herbals.

Official medicine uses comfrey externally in compresses and washes for treating burns and skin grafts, as well as to facilitate the healing of broken bones. They are also used to help relieve the swelling and pain of hemorrhoids. Fresh sliced roots and their juice are also used by physicians to help heal wounds and to stop external bleeding.

Habitat and collection: This plant is native to Europe and temperate areas of Asia, but is cultivated in the United States and Canada. It likes to grow on the banks of rivers and streams and in other areas where water is nearby. Dig up the roots in the spring, wash them well, and dry at a temperature no higher than 104°F (40°C).

Preparation and dosage: To prepare a compress, mash the fresh roots through a grinder. Soak a clean piece of cotton or gauze in the liquid and place on the wound. Cover with adhesive, plastic, or both to keep it dry. You can also place the mashed comfrey roots directly on the wound. Cover with a piece of gauze along with a bandage and protective plastic.

To prepare a decoction, add 1 tablespoon (15 g) of roots to 1 cup (250 ml) of cold water. Bring to a boil, then lower heat and simmer for 15 minutes. A standard dose is usually about $^1/_2$ cup (125 ml) 3 times a day.

Caution: **Russian scientists have found that comfrey root contains a number of poisonous substances that can be toxic to certain individuals. For this reason, we caution that internal ingestion of comfrey preparations be done *only* under the supervision of an experienced health-care professional.**

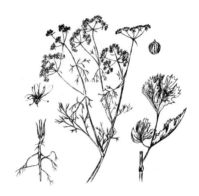

CORIANDER

Botanical name: *Coriandrum sativum.*
Family: Umbelliferae.
Also known as: Coriander seed.

A native of the eastern Mediterranean, coriander has been respected for the medicinal value of the volatile oil from its seeds as well as for its narcotic properties (when used in excess). Coriander is especially valued in China, where legend holds that it confers immortality on those who eat it. Russian peasants have traditionally used coriander seeds as a flavoring for pickles but they also use it extensively for medicinal purposes.

Herbalists recall the tale of a Russian merchant who traveled to the Mediterranean to purchase spices. Being unaccustomed to the food of the region, he became very sick but was unable to refuse the food offered him for fear of being impolite to his hosts. Finally, a local healer told him to add coriander to his food, and he became well again. Impressed with the properties of this exotic herb, he decided to buy nothing but coriander so that he could share it with the people back home. Although the legend does not reveal if his business was a success, it tells how coriander was first introduced to imperial Russia centuries ago.

Parts used: Seeds.

Actions: Analgesic, anodyne, antiseptic, antispasmodic, appetizer, carminative, cholagogue, digestive, diuretic, expectorant, stomachic, vermicide.

Medicinal virtues: A coriander infusion is recommended for liver and bladder problems. It improves appetite and digestion, imparting a soothing effect in the case of meteorism. Coriander is prescribed for expelling worms from the intestine and is also a popular bronchitis remedy. Used externally, coriander can be applied to the skin for treating rheumatism and painful joints. As a wash, it is used for cosmetic purposes and for treating eczema and neurodermatitis.

Habitat and collection: Coriander is cultivated in southern Russia, southern Europe, and North and South America. Collect the flowering heads in late summer. Remove the seeds after the umbels ripen.

Preparation and dosage: Add 1 cup (250 ml) of boiling water to 1 teaspoon (5 g) of seeds. Cover and steep for 5 minutes. Take ¹/₂ cup (125 ml) 4 times a day before meals. Or steep 10 whole fruits in 1 cup (250 ml) of hot water for 5 minutes. Take 1 cup (250 ml) twice a day.

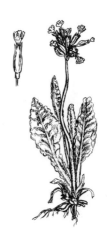

COWSLIP

Botanical name: *Primula veris.*
Family: Primulaceae.
Also known as: Primrose, butter rose,
   marsh marigold.

In Russia, this popular medicinal plant is called "prime blossom," and its use goes back thousands of years. The ancient Greeks called it *dodekateon,* or "the flower of the twelve gods" and considered it one of the healing plants of Mount Olympus, the home of the gods. Cowslip was also known among the early Slavic tribes to which many modern Russians can trace their ancestry.

In many Russian villages, it was traditional for children to collect cowslip's sweet roots in the spring. Sources of vitamin C had been depleted during the winter months, and in the early spring cowslip was a primary source of this important vitamin.

Parts used: Flowers, leaves, rootstocks.

Actions: Anodyne, antipyretic, diuretic, sedative, soporific, sudorific.

Medicinal virtues: Cowslip is an excellent sedative and can be used to treat nervous tension, nervous headache, and insomnia. It is also widely used to treat bronchitis, chills, and coughs. The leaves are valued as a source of vitamin C and other vitamins and are a helpful addition to the diet for patients with vitamin deficiencies, anemia, and general weakness.

An infusion of the roots is used as an antipyretic (febrifuge), sudorific, and expectorant for diseases of the respiratory organs, including asthma. A tea made from the flowers is a popular sedative and soporific for migraine headaches, insomnia, giddiness, and different types of neuroses. It is also used as an anodyne for joint pain (such as rheumatism) and as a diuretic to treat kidney and bladder diseases and edema. Folk healers also use an infusion of flowers to treat heart disease.

In folk medicine, the roots, leaves, and flowers together have long been popular to treat catarrhal diseases, bronchitis, whooping cough, pneumonia (as an expectorant), influenza, tonsillitis, sinusitis, and chronic constipation. Russian healers also make an ointment from cowslip leaves and flowers to treat blemishes and other skin problems.

The plant is not poisonous and can be prepared easily for home use; however, some people may be allergic to cowslip preparations, which can cause rashes and itching.

Habitat and collection: Cowslip is a perennial plant that grows in marshes and near ponds and streams in northern Russia, Europe, and North America. Dig roots together with rhizome in the fall. Wash them in cold water and set to dry. Collect the leaves during or close to the time of flowering, usually between March and May. Dry them in the sun or in an oven heated to 250°F (120°C). If dried too slowly, vitamin C may be destroyed.

Preparation and dosage: To make a decoction, add 1 teaspoon (5 g) of dried roots and rootstock to 1 cup (250 ml) of water. Bring to a boil, then reduce heat and simmer gently for 5 minutes. Take 1/2 cup (125 ml) 3 to 4 times a day. To make a leaf decoction, add 1 teaspoon (5 g) of leaves to 1/2 cup (125 ml) of water. Heat to boiling, then filter. Take 1/4 cup (62 ml) twice a day.

To prepare an infusion, add 1 cup (250 ml) of boiling water to 2 teaspoons (10 g) of flowers. Cover and steep for 15 minutes and strain. Take 1/2 cup (125 ml) 3 times a day.

CUCUMBER

Botanical name: *Cucumis sativus.*
Family: Cucurbitaceae.

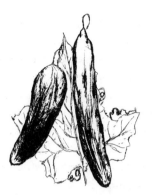

Though native to India, today's cucumber is believed to be related to plants growing in the Himalayas. Its phallic shape has long symbolized fecundity, and early Buddhist legend teaches that the first of the 60,000 offspring of King Sagara was a cucumber, who climbed to heaven on his own vine. The cucumber was an important part of the diets of those living in ancient Egypt and Palestine, and is prominently mentioned in the Bible.

Studies have shown that the cucumber is one of the world's most popular food plants, and is one of the ten most popular salad vegetables in both the United States and Russia. However, few of us realize that this refreshing vegetable possesses a respectable variety of medicinal properties, especially relating to the heart, nervous system, and eyes.

Parts used: Fruit, juice, peel, seeds, flowers.

Actions: Anesthetic, anthelmintic, antiphlogistic, aperient, diuretic.

Medicinal virtues: Over the years, the common cucumber has been researched in a number of Russian institutions. Scientists found that cucumbers stimulate the secretion of the digestive glands and increase the flow of bile. This enables the body to assimilate proteins, fat, and albumen better.

Being low in calories and high in fiber and nutrients, cucumbers are a recommended part of any weight-loss dietary regimen. Cucumbers are especially rich in potassium, which exerts a diuretic effect in cases of dropsy and edema. It is also believed to normalize the systolic actions of the heart muscle. The water and cellular tissue of the fruit have a mild purgative effect in cases of chronic constipation. It helps to purge the body of toxins and is said to have a calming effect on the nervous system.

Russian herbalists recommend cucumber juice for treating inflammation of the respiratory tract and to relieve lingering cough. It is even believed to help those who are suffering from tuberculosis.

Russian herbalists have found that decoctions made from various parts of the cucumber can treat a number of health problems. A flower decoction is used to treat malaria, while a decoction made of overripe cucumbers is good for treating liver diseases. A decoction of cucumber seeds helps to dissolve uric acid accumulations in the form of kidney and bladder stones. It is also used to reduce fever.

Cucumber juice has a tonic and bleaching effect on the skin. It is applied externally to remove freckles, blackheads, and birthmarks. It can also be used externally to soothe sores and burns. Dried cucumber powder made from seeds can be rubbed on burns, swollen areas, bedsores, skin inflammation, and other skin problems. Drops of cucumber juice directly in the eyes ease irritation.

Habitat and collection: This plant is widely cultivated in gardens throughout the world. Harvest when ripe, usually in July and August.

Preparation and dosage: As a refreshing tonic, take $1/4$ cup (60 ml) of cucumber juice 2 to 3 times a day. Prepare the juice by processing a peeled cucumber in a juicer or extractor and straining the resulting liquid.

To use as an eyewash, bring the juice to a boil and allow to cool to room temperature. Apply 1 to 2 drops to irritated eyes once a day. A course of treatment should not exceed one week.

To make a decoction, add 4 tablespoons (60 g) of crushed cucumbers with peel to 2 cups (500 ml) of boiling water. Cover and steep for 4 to 6 hours. Strain and use as a wash or cold compress.

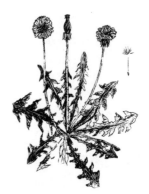

DANDELION
Botanical name: *Taraxacum officinale.*
Family: Compositae.

In times past, Russian folk herbalists called the dandelion the "elixir of life" because of its wide range of healing properties. Dandelion roots were reputed to be the favorite remedy of Panteleimon the Healer, a Russian Orthodox priest and perhaps the most famous Russian herbalist in history. The dandelion was also a favorite remedy among members of the imperial court and was used extensively by members of the royal family as a general tonic and to treat a variety of health problems.

Of particular interest was its reputed ability to make freckles disappear. In earlier times, it was considered bad for female members of the aristocracy to have too many freckles because freckles indicated that a woman would bear too many children. Although Russia no longer has an aristocracy, some Russian women still use dandelion juice to remove freckles.

In addition to its medicinal uses, some of the large-leaved varieties are cultivated for use in salads and are a popular ingredient in dandelion wine. Russian farmers often feed dandelion flowers to their rabbits.

Parts used: Leaves, flowers, roots.

Actions: Anthelmintic, antipyretic, aperient, appetizer, cholagogue, depurative, diaphoretic, diuretic, stomachic, tonic.

Medicinal virtues: Considered a "life infusion" in Russia, dandelion holds a place of honor in both folk and Russian official medicine, where it has been subject to extensive research. In official medical practice, the herb is used to treat liver and gallbladder diseases. It promotes the formation of bile and removes excess water (edema) from the body. It is an excellent tonic and depurative remedy. Dandelion promotes the dissolution of gallstones and exerts a calmative action in cases of kidney and bladder problems.

A perfect bitter remedy, dandelion increases the appetite, and the juice is a restorative remedy useful for both stomach inflammation and low acid secretion. It is also prescribed as a gentle purgative for people suffering from constipation.

In Russian folk medicine, dandelion use is also widespread. It is commonly used externally to treat skin rash, furuncles, blackheads, and other skin problems. In folk dermatology, dandelion is used to relieve itching due to eczema, neurodermatitis, and psoriasis. Both eating a salad of dandelion leaves and applying a lotion made from dandelion roots are considered effective.

Used externally, fresh dandelion juice is recommended for removing warts, corns, calluses, skin discoloration, and freckles. A lotion made from dandelion oil relieves minor burns. As an antipyretic, dandelion can help reduce fever and as a diaphoretic promotes perspiration. In rural Russia, the root extract is traditionally used to prevent miscarriages and to treat tuberculosis. Ground dandelion roots are often used to prepare a caffeine-free coffee substitute and to help eliminate poisons from the body. It is also used to treat atherosclerosis. Dandelion tea has been found effective in treating insomnia, hypochondria, and hemorrhage.

Rich in potassium, iron, and vitamins A, B_1, B_2, B_6, and C, fresh, young dandelion greens eaten in salads help prevent and treat anemia, dyspepsia with constipation, stiff joints, chronic rheumatism, and gout. If necessary, soak the leaves in cold salt water to remove the bitter taste.

Habitat and collection: The hearty dandelion is a common perennial herb that grows abundantly in lawns and meadows throughout Europe and North America. Collect the whole plant before it flowers. Harvest the leaves during flowering. Roots are best collected in the late fall when the above-ground part of the plant is dying.

Preparation and dosage: To make an infusion, add 1 cup (250 ml) of boiling water to 2 teaspoons (10 g) of fresh roots or fresh herb. Allow to steep for 10 to 15 minutes. Take $^1/_2$ to 1 cup (125 to 250 ml) of the infusion daily at room temperature. As an appetizer or as a cholagogue for treating constipation, take 1 teaspoon (5 g) of well-crushed roots and add to 1 cup (250 ml) of boiling water. Steep for 20 minutes, strain, and cool. Take $^1/_4$ cup (60 ml) 3-times daily before meals.

To prepare a decoction, add 1 tablespoon (15 g) of ground roots to 1 cup (250 ml) of water. Bring to a boil, then reduce heat and simmer gently for 15 minutes. Allow to cool for 45 minutes and strain. Take warm $^1/_3$ cup (80 ml) 3 times daily before meals.

To make dandelion juice, squeeze 1 teaspoon (5 ml) of the juice from the leaves and take 1 to 3 times a day.

The leaves can be eaten raw in summer salads.

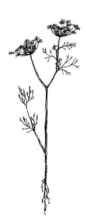

DILL
Botanical name: *Anethum graveolens.*
Family: Umbelliferae.

Dill is one of the earliest and best-known medicinal herbs in Europe. While there are not yet many books or scientific articles about the medicinal benefits of dill, there are few plants as popular in Russia today. Those who love traditional Russian borscht know that it contains a generous amount of dill, and millions of Russian cooks use dill when making pickles. For many families, preserving foods with dill is crucial to maintaining health during the winter months when fresh fruits and vegetables are not available. For that reason, dill is often linked with the preservation of life and health. It is only recently that Russian scientists have discovered that dill contains special types of acids, which explain its medicinal properties.

Parts used: Aerial parts, seeds.

Actions: Antispasmodic, antitussive, calmative, carminative, diuretic, galactagogue, stomachic.

Medicinal virtues: A tincture made from dried, powdered dill seeds is used as a diuretic and helps stop coughing. Nursing mothers are sometimes advised to take an infusion of powdered seeds to promote the flow of milk. It is also recommended as a mild calmative for people suffering from insomnia and nervous tension. Fifteen to twenty drops of a tincture of dill seed in 1/4 cup (60 ml) of cold water is often prescribed to treat early symptoms of hypertonia, or abnormal tension of arteries or muscles. A decoction made of dill is prescribed for gastritis with reduced acidity. It also assists in expelling gas from the intestines and strengthens and stimulates the stomach in general.

Externally, dill is used in cold compresses or as an eyewash for inflammatory eye diseases like iritis (inflammation of the iris), iridocyclitis (irritation of the iris and ciliary body of the eye), and conjunctivitis (irritation of the mucous membrane that lines the eyelid).

Preparation and dosage: To make an infusion, steep 2 teaspoons (10 g) of seeds in 1 cup (250 ml) of boiling water for 10 to 12 minutes. Strain liquid and take 1/2 cup (125 ml) at a time 2 or 3 times a day.

To prepare a decoction, pour 1 cup (250 ml) of hot water into a pot containing 3 1/2 tablespoons (50 g) of dried crushed herb. Cover pot and boil over a low flame for 15 minutes. Cool at room temperature for 45 minutes. Filter and add water to bring up the level of the water until it reaches 1 cup (250 ml) again. Take 1/3 cup (80 ml) 3 times a day before meals. Take 1/2 cup (125 ml) of a dill decoction before meals to relieve flatulence.

ELDER

Botanical name: *Sambucus nigra*.
Family: Caprifoliaceae.
Also known as: Black elder,
European elder.

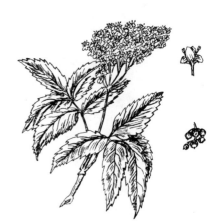

A common hedge tree found in eastern Russia and other parts of northern Europe, early Russians believed that the elder was the home of a tree spirit, usually in the form of an old woman. In medieval times, elder wood was used to cure toothache, interrupt epileptic fits, remove poison from metal vessels, and guarantee that the person who cultivated it would die in his or her own home.

Parts used: Bark, flowers, fruit, leaves.

Actions: Aperient, diaphoretic, diuretic, emetic, purgative, vulnerary.

Medicinal virtues: In official Russian herbal medicine, an extract of elder flowers is used to treat chronic inflammation of the respiratory tract, including bronchitis, pneumonia, asthma, and other lung problems. It is also used to treat colds by raising the body temperature and promoting perspiration. A warm extract of elder flowers is recommended as a gargle for people with chronic tonsillitis.

In folk medicine, an infusion of elder flowers has traditionally been used to treat rheumatism, gout, and kidney problems, as well as sinusitis and hay-fever symptoms.

In folk dermatology, elder flower infusions are used as an antiseptic wash for skin problems, including chronic eczema, psoriasis, seborrhea, dermatitis, and hair loss. In these cases, an extract from elder flowers is rubbed on the affected area. Flower extracts also help reduce inflammation around muscles and joints. A combination of elder flowers and chamomile flowers used in equal proportions are boiled in water and used as a compress.

Preparations made from the young leaves are an effective remedy for arthritis, rheumatic complaints, arteriosclerosis, and diabetes. Leaves are also used to make an external ointment good for treating eye and ear diseases, toothache, and bone pain. Leaves applied directly to the skin are also used for burns, furuncles, skin irritations, and open wounds. For these purposes, steam the leaves, spread in a single layer on a dry surface, and pat gently with a paper towel to remove excess moisture.

Elderberries are never to be eaten raw, and the fresh juice cannot be used.* Cook the fresh berries in boiling water for 5 to 10 minutes, whether for eating or for making juice. Dried berries should be boiled for 15 minutes.

An infusion made of spring leaves and autumn berries mixed with honey is used in folk medicine to cure chronic constipation. An extract made of elderberries and young shoots is recommended to treat kidney problems accompanied by edema. It increases the production of urine and helps to eliminate excess water from the body.

Elder flowers and berries can be used to make cake fillings, jam, candies, and jelly. These preparations are all mildly laxative and are suitable for people with irritated or inflamed intestines.

Habitat and collection: Elder is native to northern Europe, including Great Britain, and western Asia. Elder blooms from May until June, when the flowers can be collected and dried in a shady place. The berries ripen from June through August and are best collected in August and September.

Preparation and dosage: To make an infusion, add 1 cup (250 ml) boiling water to 2 teaspoons (10 g) of flowers. Allow to steep for 10 minutes and then strain. Drink the infusion 2 to 3 times a day.

To prepare a decoction for treating kidney diseases, rheumatism, and podagra, add 1 tablespoon (15 g) of crushed, dried herb to 1 cup (250 ml) of hot water. Heat to a boil then simmer for 15 minutes. Allow to cool for 45 minutes and filter. Take warm ⅓ to ½ cup (80 to 125 ml) 2 to 3 times daily before meals.

To make an ointment, British herbalist David Hoffmann recommends taking 3 parts of fresh leaves and heating with 6 parts of petroleum jelly until the leaves are crisp. Strain and store in a covered container at room temperature.

Caution: **Do not use the species of elder called *Sambucus racemosa*; despite some medicinal virtues of the berries, their seeds are poisonous.**

———

* This pertains to the European species, *Sambucus nigra*. The North American species, *S. canadensis,* produces edible berries, however.

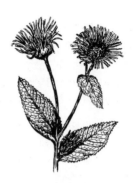

ELECAMPANE
Botanical name: *Inula helenium.*
Family: Compositae.
Also known as: Elfdock, horse elder.

Elecampane is one of the oldest herbs in the Russian tradition. It is called "ninepowers" in the Russian language, while the Ukrainians know it as "wonderful power," attesting to its myriad applications. Although it is found growing wild throughout the countryside, many Russians cultivate elecampane in their gardens.

Reference to this herb can be traced to the seventeenth century, when the court physician to Czar Michael Fedorovich prescribed this herb for the czar and his family. An herbal dated at 1672 states that "The root of the Ninepowers should be crushed and mixed with raw honey . . . and be taken in the morning and the evening. It will calm down coughing and expel any thick phlegm inside the throat. The same root cooked in wine and sweetened with sugar is good, and when taken internally helps people breathe easier."

Parts used: Flowers, leaves, rootstocks.

Actions: Anthelmintic, antibacterial, antiphlogistic, cholagogue, digestive, diuretic, emmenagogue, expectorant, hemostatic, stimulant, stomachic, sudorific, tonic, vulnerary.

Medicinal virtues: Elecampane has a wide range of therapeutic applications. A decoction made from elecampane root is often prescribed as an antiphlogistic and hemostatic for treating problems of the gastrointestinal tract. It increases stomach and intestinal secretions thus stimulating the appetite and improving digestion. It is also used to relieve diarrhea and hemorrhoids. A decoction is used by official herbalists to treat painful or irregular menstruation. It is recommended for giddiness, headaches, heart palpitations, and epilepsy.

A root decoction is recommended for treating bronchial asthma, bronchitis (with frequent expectoration), whooping cough, tuberculosis, and pneumonia. It is also used to reduce high blood pressure and to expel intestinal worms. A clinically tested and approved elecampane preparation, which is marketed under the name Alanton, is prescribed in Russia to stimulate blood circulation in the stomach and to accelerate the healing of stomach ulcers. Decoctions are also used externally for treating inflammation of the gums and as a wash for relieving itchy skin.

In folk medicine, elecampane infusions are recommended for treating nervousness, duodenal ulcers, goiter, and high blood pressure. Fresh leaves are used to treat sores and scrofula, a type of tuberculosis adenitis.

Habitat and collection: A hearty plant, elecampane is found by roadsides and in waste places throughout western Russia, northern Europe, and much of the United States. The root can be harvested from early September through the end of October.

Preparation and dosage: To make a decoction, place 2 tablespoons (30 g) of roots into a pot and add 1 cup (250 ml) of hot water. Cover loosely, bring to a boil, then reduce heat and simmer gently for 30 minutes (a water banya is recommended for this procedure if you have access to one). Strain. Take warm ½ cup (125 ml) 2 to 3 times daily 1 hour before meals.

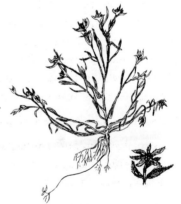

EVERLASTING
Botanical name: *Gnaphalium uliginosum.*
Family: Compositae.
Also known as: Cudweed, low cudweed,
  marsh cudweed, life everlasting.

Everlasting, known in Russia as "the immortalizer," is one of the oldest Russian herbs. Early folk healers in many areas of imperial Russia used it for centuries, and references to using cudweed can be found in several early handwritten herbals. The most common reports speak of cudweed as a remedy for treating wounds and open sores, and folk healers often used cudweed preparations to relieve stomach pain. It also was known by the name "toad's herb" because it treated quinsy and tonsillitis, which were known collectively by the slang expression "toad."

Everlasting traces its popularity more through word of mouth than from old Russian herbal books. This oral tradition eventually attracted the attention of mainstream Russian physicians, and the first serious scientific research into the medicinal properties of this herb began in the early 1930s. Before the outbreak of the Second World War, everlasting was adopted by official Russian medicine as a recommended medical treatment.

Parts used: Aerial parts.

Actions: Anodyne, anticatarrhal, antiseptic, astringent, calmative, diuretic, hemostatic, vasodilator, vulnerary.

Medicinal virtues: Everlasting preparations are used widely both in folk and official medicine in Russia. When taken internally as an infusion, everlasting is useful in relieving early symptoms of hypertension and can reduce stenocardia and heart palpitations. It reduces arterial pressure and dilates the blood vessels. Infusions are also used to treat headaches, insomnia, nervous excitability, asthma, diabetes, and as a gargle to treat tonsillitis and quinsy.

Both infusions and decoctions are considered effective for treating stomach and duodenal ulcers as well as for relieving symptoms of gastritis and diarrhea. As a hemostatic, an everlasting infusion or decoction is used to stop internal bleeding, especially in the intestines or the uterus. A decoction is also prescribed as a wash for healing abrasions of the uterus and vaginitis. Used as a poultice, an everlasting decoction is also good for stopping external bleeding.

An alcohol or oil extract or infusion of this herb heals old sores, wounds, chemical and thermal burns, trophic ulcers, dermatomycosis, and wet eczema. An oil extract is reputed to prevent balding if rubbed into the scalp.

Habitat and collection: Everlasting grows in damp soil in Russia, Canada, and in northern regions of the United States. Collect in August, and dry in a shady place.

Preparation and dosage: To prepare an infusion, add 1 cup (250 ml) of boiling water to 1 tablespoon (15 g) of dried herb. Steep for 10 minutes. Strain. Take 1 cup (250 ml) 3 times a day.

To make a decoction, place 2 tablespoons (30 g) of dried herb in 1 cup (250 ml) of hot water. Boil for 15 minutes, cool at room temperature for 45 minutes, and strain, remembering to squeeze the last drops of the decoction through the strainer. Drink $\frac{1}{2}$ cup (125 ml) 3 times a day after meals. May be taken for 1 to 2 months.

To treat hypertension, make the same decoction but use it as a foot bath. Place 9 ounces (250 g) of the herb in $1\frac{1}{4}$ gallons (5 liters) of water heated to 90 to 95°F (32 to 35°C). Let stand for 30 minutes. Take this foot bath once a day, a half hour before bedtime.

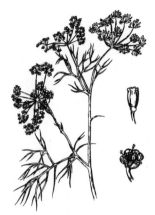

FENNEL

Botanical name: *Foeniculum vulgare.*
Family: Umbelliferae.
Also known as: Large fennel, sweet fennel,
   wild fennel.

Fennel shares a similar name in most European languages (in Russian, it is pronounced "FEN-hel"), and its medicinal use goes back to ancient Greece and Rome. Renowned physicians like Hippocrates, Diascorides, and Galen were acquainted with fennel. Of course, Russian folk healers used fennel before Greek manuscripts reached the Slavic world. As with many other ancient herbs, the modern knowledge we now possess is the culmination of many herbal traditions over the centuries.

Parts used: Ripe seeds, oil of seeds.

Actions: Antispasmodic, aromatic, carminative, diuretic, expectorant, galactagogue, hydragogue, stimulant, stomachic.

Medicinal virtues: Fennel seeds contain large amounts of anethole, a volatile oil that produces an antispasmodic effect on the smooth muscles of the intestines, which inhibits a buildup of intestinal gas. The seeds also help maintain the tone of the stomach muscles and help fight intestinal tract infections.

In the Russian herbal tradition, fennel is prescribed to relieve abdominal cramps, colic, meteorism, bronchitis with mucus, phlegm that is difficult to discharge, and edema. In Russia, fennel is used as a gargle to cure hoarseness and cough. Preparations made from fennel seeds stimulate the flow of milk in nursing mothers and are believed to help regulate menstruation. Fennel also has some purgative and diuretic properties.

Russian folk healers rub fennel seed oil on sore muscles and areas prone to rheumatism. Some sources recommend using cold compresses of a fennel decoction combined with taking a fennel infusion internally to treat eczema and neurodermatitis, while an infusion prepared as a cold compress soothes conjunctivitis and inflammation of the eyelids. In addition, fennel is recommended as an ingredient in more complex herbal preparations to treat these same health problems.

In some areas of south Russia, fennel leaves are used as spices. Juicy leaves and young umbels are canned, while fresh leaves are used in baking.

Habitat and collection: Fennel grows wild in southern Russia, Belarus, and Ukraine, but is also widely cultivated throughout Europe, Canada, and the United States. The best time to collect the plant is just before flowering. Leaves can be used fresh, or they can also be frozen or infused with oil or vinegar.

Preparations and dosage: To make an infusion, pour 1 cup (250 ml) of boiling water into a container with 1 tablespoon (15 g) of dried ground fennel seeds. Allow to stand for 10 minutes. Strain. Take 1/2 cup (125 ml) 2 to 3 times a day. Honey may also be added for better taste.

To prepare a fennel cleansing milk to treat oily skin, heat 1/2 cup (125 ml) of buttermilk and add 2 tablespoons (30 g) of fennel seeds. Cook gently for 30 minutes and allow to stand for 2 hours. Strain and place in a closed container. Refrigerate for no longer than 1 week. Wash the face once a day with the mixture.

Chew fennel seeds as a good breath freshener.

Caution: **If taken internally, large amounts of fennel seed oil can be toxic to the liver and may cause epileptic-like convulsions. However, small amounts used as a flavoring, as well as fennel seeds in an infusion as described above, are safe.**

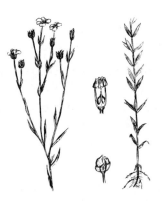

FLAX

Botanical name: *Linum usitatissimum.*
Family: Linaceae.
Also known as: Linseed.

Humans have used the flax plant for thousands of years. Linen cloth made of flax was found in Stone Age settlements dated before 4000 B.C.E. Flaxseed (linseed) oil has long been prized by artists who use the oil in their paints. The oil has become popular for massaging the chests of bronchitis sufferers and is a source of vitamin E and essential fatty acids.

Part used: Ripe seeds.

Actions: Anodyne, anthelmintic, antiphlogistic, demulcent, digestive, emollient, laxative, purgative, vulnerary.

Medicinal virtues: Infusions and decoctions made from flaxseeds are used as an antiphlogistic to treat inflammations of the mucous membranes of the gastrointestinal tract, including stomach and duodenal ulcers, gastritis, chronic colitis, and enterocolitis. It is also recommended in cases of food poisoning. A decoction from seeds regulates the secretory and motor functions of the large and small intestines. Infusions and decoctions are prescribed to treat inflammations of the respiratory tract, including bronchitis and quinsy.

An infusion of seeds is used externally as a cold compress or a fomentation to treat furuncles and other inflammatory diseases of the skin. It is also good as a gargle for mouth sores and other inflammations. Infusions are also recommended as enemas for treating colitis and as douches for treating gynecological infections.

In Russian folk medicine, both infusions and decoctions of seeds are valued for their anthelmintic properties and as a laxative to treat intestinal diseases, including chronic constipation. They are also recommended for gallbladder and kidney problems.

Flaxseeds are a part of a dietary program to treat arteriosclerosis and an approved medication made from the seeds, and known as Linetol, is prescribed by Russian physicians to help lower serum cholesterol. Flaxseeds are also recommended as part of a weight-loss regimen. A powder made from seeds helps to heal burns and skin abscesses. Dry seeds can be heated and applied externally to sore muscles and joints.

Flaxseed oil can be used as a massage oil on the chest to relieve symptoms of chronic bronchitis. The oil is also taken internally to treat gallstones.

Habitat and collection: Flax is found growing wild along railroad beds and roadsides throughout Europe and North America, but it is also widely cultivated. Harvest the seedpods in September.

Preparation and dosage: To make an infusion, take 3 tablespoons (45 g) of well-crushed seeds and add to 3 cups (750 ml) of boiling water. Steep for 15 minutes. Cool and strain. Take ¹/₂ cup (125 ml) 3 times a day during meals. To make an infusion for chronic constipation, add 1 teaspoon (5 g) of seeds to 1 cup of boiling water. Cool and strain. Take entire cup before bedtime.

To make a cold infusion, add 1 to 3 tablespoons (15 to 45 g) of crushed seeds to 1 cup (250 ml) of cold water. Allow to stand for 2 to 3 hours, stirring every 30 minutes. Strain. Take ¹/₄ cup (62 ml) 3 times a day.

To prepare a decoction, add 1 tablespoon (15 g) of ripe seeds to 1 quart (1 liter) of boiling water. Continue to boil on a low flame until half the liquid remains. Strain. Take ¹/₂ cup (125 ml) 4 times a day.

Caution: Immature seeds (generally those collected before September) can cause poisoning.

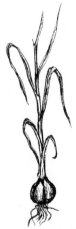

GARLIC
Botanical name: *Allium sativum.*
Family: Liliaceae.

In ancient times, Russians believed that wearing amulets made of garlic would protect them from infectious diseases, which were believed to be caused by witchcraft or evil spirits. Although Russians do not wear necklaces made of garlic anymore, garlic is one of the best-known and most widely used herbs in Russia today and is prized for its antibacterial, virucidal, and antiparasitic properties.

Garlic has long been used as both an antibiotic and an antiseptic. During the Second World War, Russian doctors and medics used garlic in the field to treat bullet, shrapnel, and other war-related wounds. It was held to have prevented many cases of battle-related diseases like gangrene and sepsis. During the war, garlic even became known by Allied troops as "Russian penicillin."

Garlic has been a subject of scientific research for many years. In the late 1920s Russian medical researcher B. P. Tokin discovered that crushed garlic cloves contain the enzyme alliinase, which produces an aromatic volatile oil known scientifically today as diallyl disulfide. Dr. Tokin found that this oil could kill harmful microorganisms. When a mashed garlic clove is placed under a glass dome with cultured bacteria or fungi, the microorganisms die within minutes. He discovered that this oil is also present in onions, but garlic offers a stronger concentration. Scientists have since found that garlic compounds can inhibit both the growth of cancerous tumors and malignant cells in general. For this reason garlic is an important part of a holistic approach to treating cancer.

Russian folk healers have long recommended eating one clove of raw garlic a day, preferably at dinnertime. Those who find eating raw garlic disagreeable can add it to salads or mix it with some salt and chopped tomatoes and spread it on a slice of dark Russian rye bread. Many people in America take deodorized garlic supplements in capsules, although Russian herbalists recommend ingesting garlic in its natural form.

Parts used: Bulb.

Actions: Analgesic, antibacterial, antibiotic, antiparasitic, antiseptic, depurative, diaphoretic, diuretic, stimulant, vasodilator, vermicide, virucidal.

Medicinal virtues: Garlic stimulates the activity of the body's digestive organs, and Russian official medicine considers garlic preparations effective for treating a wide variety of digestive health complaints including lack of tone in the intestines, poor digestion, colitis, enterocolitis, and problems related to the presence of putrefactive bacteria in the intestines. It is also used to help expel parasites (especially pinworms) from the intestine, as well as to stimulate proper liver and gallbladder function.

Garlic is an effective remedy in treating bronchitis and catarrh and is used to reduce excess blood sugar. It is also considered an overall heart strengthener and is prescribed for patients suffering from arteriosclerosis and high blood pressure. Russian doctors also recommend garlic for people who have been exposed to lead poisoning.

Russian folk herbalists maintain that garlic is a good preventive against colds, flu, and other diseases caused by viruses. To treat coughs, bronchitis, or sinus problems, they recommend taking 1 tablespoon (15 g) of crushed garlic mixed with honey 2 to 3 times a day. Folk herbalists also use garlic to treat migraine headaches and insomnia. Russian folk herbalists have long used the steam from boiling garlic cloves to help heal skin ulcers and infected skin wounds. To treat skin problems such as corns, they recommend that raw garlic cloves be placed on a corn for 12 to 18 hours. After this treatment, the corn often goes away, although the patient may experience pain for another 12 hours.

Habitat and collection: Garlic is cultivated in gardens throughout the world and thrives best in sandy or loamy soil. When planted in early spring, the bulbs are usually ready to harvest in August or September.

Preparation and dosage: To make a garlic infusion, take 1 teaspoon (5 g) of raw crushed garlic and add to 2 cups (500 ml) of preboiled water that has been left to cool for 10 minutes. Allow to stand for 1 hour. Take 1 cup (250 ml) 3 times daily before meals. As an alternative, mix 2 ounces (approximately 50 g) of crushed raw garlic with 2 cups (500 ml) of sour clotted milk. Allow to stand for 12 hours. Take 1 tablespoon (15 ml) 3 to 4 times daily before meals.

To prepare a garlic tincture, crush 7 ounces (200 g) of peeled garlic cloves and place in a glass bottle containing 1 quart (1 liter) of 90-proof alcohol spirits. Close the bottle and allow to stand for 14 days at approximately 85°F (28°C). Take 15 to 20 drops 2 to 3 times daily for treating poor digestion, colitis, hypertonia, and atherosclerosis.

Folk herbalists often recommend eating two to three cloves of garlic whenever you are exposed to colds or flu.

Caution: **People suffering from kidney problems should avoid garlic remedies because garlic can irritate the kidneys.**

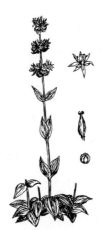

YELLOW GENTIAN
Botanical name: *Gentiana lutea.*
Family: Gentianaceae.
Also known as: Gentian, bitterwort,
    pale gentian.

It is said that the family name (Gentianaceae) for this herb traces its origin to the ancient Greek King Gentius, an accomplished healer who used herbs from this family to heal members of his court. The Russian name of this herb (translated in English as "bittering yellow") refers more to its bitter taste. Monks often added it to liquors they made in their monasteries, which were often consumed as appetizers before large banquets. Although many of the original recipes have been lost over the centuries, yellow gentian is still used in the preparation of some liquors in Russia today.

Yellow gentian is listed in the *Russian Red Book* of rare, endangered herbs and plants, and its collection in the wild is prohibited by law. Fortunately, this herb is easy to cultivate, and many Russians give it a prominent place in their family herb garden. Russian scientists began investigating the chemical and medicinal properties of yellow gentian in 1955. It is now considered an important herb of the pharmacopeia of official Russian medicine.

Parts used: Roots.

Actions: Appetizer, cholagogue, febrifuge, refrigerant, stomachic, tonic.

Medicinal virtues: The most popular use of yellow gentian is to improve gastrointestinal function, such as increasing appetite and aiding digestion. However, it is also recognized as a safe treatment for a wide variety of more serious common gastrointestinal problems like stomachache, heartburn, indigestion, catarrhal gastritis (especially when accompanied by diarrhea), and vomiting. It is also regarded as an immune booster, because it raises the white blood cell count.

Russian herbalists use a decoction of the root externally to disinfect wounds. When placed on open wounds and inflammations, the fresh leaves act as a refrigerant, and when soaked in cold water make a soothing foot bath. In times past, folk healers used preparations made with yellow gentian root to treat such deadly diseases as plague, tuberculosis, and malaria.

Habitat and collection: Yellow gentian is a perennial that grows in pastures and mountain meadows throughout Europe and Asia Minor, although it is widely cultivated in Europe and North America. Dig up the roots in the autumn. The leaves can be collected at any time.

Preparation and dosage: To make a decoction, add $1/2$ teaspoon ($2^1/2$ g) of dried roots to 1 cup (250 ml) of water. Boil the mixture for 3 to 4 minutes, and allow to cool. Take 1 tablespoon (15 ml) every 2 hours at least 30 minutes before meals.

To prepare an infusion, add $1/2$ teaspoon ($2^1/2$ g) of dried roots to 1 cup (250 ml) of boiling water. Steep until cool. Strain and add $3/4$ cup (200 ml) of brandy. Take 1 teaspoon (5 ml) 3 to 4 times a day at least 30 minutes before mealtime.

To make a cold extract, soak $1/2$ teaspoon (5 g) of dried roots in 1 cup (250 ml) of water at room temperature for 2 hours. Take 1 cup over the course of the day.

To prepare a root decoction, add 2 cups (500 ml) of cold water to 1 tablespoon (15 g) of dried roots. Bring to a boil and simmer for 10 minutes. Filter. Take $1/2$ cup (125 ml) 3 times a day.

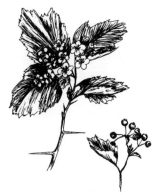

HAWTHORN

Botanical name: *Crataegus oxyacantha.*
Family: Rosaceae.
Also known as: May tree, whitethorn,
  may bush.

The Russian name for this plant is *boyarinya*, loosely translated as "your honor, lady landowner." To Russians this plant suggested a rich and inaccessible lady because it has attractive red fruits protected by sharp thorns. The name may also derive from the days of the czars, when only wealthy landowners and members of the court wore brightly colored clothing, and hawthorn berries were commonly used to dye cloth red. In Old Russian, the same word is used for *red* and *beautiful,* and red was favored by female members of the landed gentry.

More than forty different kinds of hawthorn are currently being studied in Russian medical institutes. In addition to the variety of hawthorn mentioned here, another type, *Crateagus sanguinea,* has similar medicinal properties and is used the same way.

Parts used: Flowers, fruit.

Actions: Antispasmodic, cardiac, sedative, vasodilator.

Medicinal virtues: Preparations of hawthorn are considered very powerful and have long been used to treat a variety of heart-related diseases, including inflammation of the cardiac muscular tissue (myocarditis), irregular heartbeat, and narrowing of the blood vessels. Hawthorn is also used to treat symptoms of chest discomfort, dizziness, shortness of breath, and nervousness and is believed to help maintain normal body metabolism. Because hawthorn normalizes sleep, it is often prescribed to speed up the healing process after illness or operation. The long-term use of this herb has been found to lower blood pressure and serum cholesterol, so it is often recommended for patients suffering from hypertension.

Habitat and collection: Hawthorn grows as either a shrub or tree and is native to Europe, northern Africa, and western Asia. It is often cultivated in Russia and North America as an ornamental. Because the plant blooms at different latitudes, the flowers can be harvested right after blooming, while berries are harvested upon ripening later in the summer.

Preparation and dosage: To make an infusion, add 1 cup (250 ml) of boiling water to 1 tablespoon (15 g) of dried flowers. Cover and steep for 10 to 15 minutes and filter. Take ¹/₂ cup (125 ml) 3 times a day before meals, sweetened with honey if desired.

A decoction is prepared by adding 1 tablespoon (15 g) of crushed fruits to 1 cup (250 ml) of water. Boil over a low flame for 10 minutes, then let stand for another 30 minutes. Take ¹/₃ to ¹/₂ cup (80 to 125 ml) 2 to 3 times a day a half hour before mealtimes. If desired, it can also be sweetened with honey. The decoction can be refrigerated in a tightly covered glass or porcelain container for 24 hours.

In addition to the homemade remedies mentioned here, commercial preparations made from hawthorn berries are easily available in natural food stores.

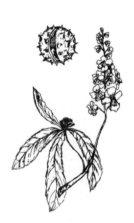

Horse Chestnut
Botanical name: *Aesculus hippocastanum.*
Family: Hippocastanaceae.
Also known as: Buckeye, Spanish chestnut.

The horse chestnut tree is native to the Caucasus and the Balkans and was introduced to the rest of Europe during the sixteenth century. Because the fruits were fed to horses and cattle as both a food and perhaps as a medicinal, the name horse chestnut has remained. This distinctive tree is planted as an ornamental throughout northern Europe and many parts of North America.

Parts used: Bark, flowers, fruit, leaves, seeds.

Actions: Antipyretic, astringent, expectorant, hemostatic, stomachic, vaso-constrictor.

Medicinal virtues: The horse chestnut enjoys a wide range of therapeutic applications in both official and folk-healing traditions. Russian herbalists recommend decoctions made of the bark and fruit of horse chestnut for chronic digestive disorders, as well as for normalizing deficient bile flow. It can also be taken internally to relieve hemorrhoids and blood vessel spasms and to constrict the blood vessels. Herbalists consider hot infusions and extracts of this plant to be among the best remedies for treating varicose veins and phlebitis. Decoctions are also prescribed to treat podagra and rheumatism and to relieve symptoms of sciatica, neuralgia, sciatic neuritis, and thrombophlebitis.

Bark and fruit decoctions are popular for treating inflammations of the respiratory tract, including catarrh of the lungs, catarrh of the nasal mucosa, and cough. In folk medicine, decoctions of the bark mixed with branches, flowers, and seeds are used to treat hemorrhoids, joint inflammation, and inflammation of the gallbladder. This combination is also considered a good hemostatic for women suffering from uterine hemorrhage (metrorrhagia). Bark baths reduce inflammation in the muscles and are considered useful for treating symptoms of neuralgia.

Habitat and collection: This tree is commonly cultivated in Europe, the United States, and parts of Canada. The chestnuts are harvested from the tree early in the fall.

Preparation and dosage: To prepare an infusion, add 1 cup (250 ml) of boiling water to 1 tablespoon (15 g) of dried fruit. Steep for 10 to 15 minutes and filter. Drink 3 times a day.

To make a decoction of leaves and fruit, add 1 teaspoon (5 g) of dried leaves and 1 teaspoonful (5 g) of dried fruit to 1 cup (250 ml) of boiling water. Continue to boil for 30 minutes. Strain. Add additional water to make up for the water that evaporated. During the first 2 days, take 1 teaspoon (5 ml) once a day, then 1 teaspoon (5 ml) 2 to 3 times a day after meals. For treating varicose veins, continue this regimen for 2 to 8 weeks (no longer than 12 weeks); for hemorrhoids, follow the regimen for 1 to 4 weeks.

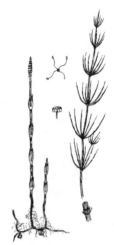

HORSETAIL

Botanical name: *Equisetum arvense.*
Family: Equisetaceae.
Also known as: Shave grass, horsetail grass,
    horsetail weed.

Horsetail is found throughout Russia. Archaeological excavations reveal that this plant was popular many centuries ago as a healing herb. An old Russian manuscript refers to a "coughing disease" that affected a beautiful young maiden in the town of Ryazan. The situation was so bad that "blood dripped out of her mouth," a probable reference to tuberculosis. The story describes how a local healer took some "shave grass which was like sand and stones and gave it to the maiden. The sand and stones were placed on her chest, and the cough ceased."

This description accurately conveys the abrasive nature of horsetail grass, which is rich in silica. In times past, horsetail was used to clean pots and pans. Although modern abrasives have replaced horsetail as a pot cleaner, millions of Russians still use it regularly as a medicinal herb.

Parts used: Young green shoots (stems).

Actions: Antiphlogistic, coagulant, diuretic, germifuge, vermicide, vulnerary.

Medicinal virtues: Horsetail is used as a diuretic to quickly reduce edema in individuals suffering from heart trouble and diseases of the kidneys. In addition to its rapid action, its effects are often prolonged. It is also recommended for inflammatory diseases of the urinary tract.

Horsetail preparations are recommended for treating atherosclerosis of the blood vessels of the heart and brain. It is also able to treat slow-healing ulcers, purulent wounds, and furuncles. In Russia, cold decoctions of this herb are often used as a gargle for inflammations of the mucous membranes of the mouth and throat and as an eyewash to treat conjunctivitis. Horsetail decoctions are often used as a cold compress on the face before bedtime to treat oily skin. The properties of this herb as a coagulant make it a recommended remedy to decrease menstrual and hemorrhoidal bleeding. Fresh horsetail juice is often prescribed as part of a complex herbal treatment of tuberculosis and is used by herbalists to treat anemia resulting from bleeding stomach ulcers.

Unfortunately, there have been no published studies in Russian medical journals about horsetail's well-known ability to stimulate the immune system. However, even a short look at the chemical and biological properties of this herb may offer promise to patients suffering from HIV infection and AIDS-related health problems.

Habitat and collection: In Russia, horsetail grows nearly everywhere that grass does, and June and July are the best months to collect it. The stems can be tied together in bundles and dried in a ventilated area.

Preparation and dosage: To make a decoction, put 2 tablespoons (30 g) of crushed fresh herb or 1 teaspoon (5 g) of dried herb in a pot. Slowly add 1 cup (250 ml) of boiling water, cover loosely, and continue to boil at low heat for 25 to 30 minutes. Allow to cool at room temperature for 10 minutes. Filter. Take $^1/_3$ to $^1/_2$ cup (80 to 125 ml) 3 to 4 times a day 1 hour after meals. Do not take horsetail for longer than 1 month. After a month, do not use for 1 week; after a week, you can safely take horsetail decoctions for another month.

To make fresh horsetail juice, collect the herb early in the morning before the dew dries. Wash in cold water, and allow it to dry for a few minutes. Pour some boiling water onto the herb, and immediately grind it in a food grinder or processor. Filter and separate the juice. Boil the juice over a low flame for 2 to 3 minutes, remove from heat, and allow to cool. Store in the refrigerator in a tightly closed container for up to a week. Take 1 tablespoon (15 ml) 3 to 4 times a day after meals.

To prepare a horsetail gargle, boil 1 cup (250 ml) of water and allow it to cool to room temperature. Put 3 heaping teaspoons (20 g) of the fresh herb, cut into small pieces, in a pot with a lid. Pour the cooled water into the pot. Cover and allow to stand for 24 hours. Use it as a gargle or for cold compresses.

To make an infusion, steep 4 tablespoons (60 g) of dried horsetail in 1 cup (250 ml) of water. Take $^1/_2$ cup (125 ml) 3 times a day 1 hour after meals.

To make a refreshing footbath, put 2 to $3^1/_2$ ounces (75 to 100 g) of fresh herb in a large pot. Pour 5 to 6 quarts (5 to 6 liters) of hot water into the pot and boil for 5 to 7 minutes. Allow to cool to a temperature of 98°F (35 to 36°C). Use 2 to 3 times a week for 20 minutes per application.

Caution: Although regarded as safe in small dosages, horsetail preparations can be toxic when consumed excessively.

ICELAND MOSS

Botanical name: *Cetraria islandica.*
Family: Parmeliaceae.
Also known as: Iceland lichen.

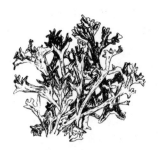

Iceland moss is not a moss, but a lichen. Aside from Iceland, it is a common plant in northern Europe and Canada. It has attracted much attention from Russian scientists during this century due to its ability to help the body heal itself from a wide range of pulmonary diseases and gastrointestinal disorders.

Parts used: Whole lichen.

Actions: Antibacterial, antiemetic, antiphlogistic, appetizer, calmative, cholagogue, demulcent, emollient, mucilaginous, purgative, tonic, vulnerary.

Medicinal virtues: In official Russian medicine, a decoction made from this lichen is prescribed for a wide variety of respiratory problems, including chronic bronchitis, chronic bronchial catarrh, bronchial asthma, and whooping cough. Because it can dissolve mucous congestion and hinders the growth of *Tubercle bacillus*, it is often prescribed for patients suffering from both pneumonia and tuberculosis.

Iceland moss has both a purgative and emollient effect on the gastrointestinal tract. It is often recommended for patients with stomach problems, including stomach and duodenal ulcers and catarrh. It also regulates the production of gastric acid. Because of its mucilage content, Iceland moss helps treat both chronic constipation and diarrhea.

When mashed and mixed with water, Iceland moss is recommended for treating sores, burns, purulent rashes, and boils. Physicians also recommend it as a vaginal douche because of its emollient and demulcent properties.

Habitat and collection: Iceland moss grows in cool damp places. Gather the lichen between May and September. Clean thoroughly and dry in a sunny or shady place.

Preparation and dosage: When a decoction of Iceland moss cools it becomes thick and viscid. To prepare a decoction, add 2 teaspoons (10 g) of plant to 2 cups (500 ml) of cold water. Bring to a boil, filter, and allow to cool. Drink the 2 cups during the day. You can also add 3 cups (750 ml) of boiling water to a pot containing $1^1/_2$ to $3^1/_2$ tablespoons (20 to 50 grams) of the plant. Boil for 30 minutes and allow to cool. Drink throughout the day.

To make an infusion (to be used primarily as a purgative), add 7 to 14 tablespoons (100 to 200 g) of plant to 1 to 2 quarts (1 to 2 liters) of cold water. Steep for 24 hours. Strain the infusion. Take 3 times a day before meals over a period of 10 to 15 days; take just enough of the infusion to produce its purgative effects. Usually between ¹/₃ and ¹/₂ cup (80 to 125 ml) is sufficient. In addition, herbalists recommend that a course of treatment last no longer than two weeks since prolonged use can irritate the gastrointestinal tract.

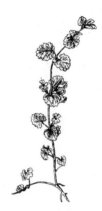

GROUND IVY
Botanical name: *Nepeta hederacea.*
Family: Labiatae.
Also known as: Alehoof, catsfoot, haymaids.

Ground ivy is a common plant in Russia and other parts of Europe and can often be found growing in hedges and waste areas throughout the continent. A hearty plant, it resembles true ivy and is known for crowding out other species. This plant was best known in centuries past for clarifying beer before hops became used for this purpose.

When I was a schoolboy, I often spent my vacation at my grandmother's house in a small town in the south of Russia. One day, after running around in the woods in shorts, I got a skin infection on one of my legs below the knee, which soon broke out in painful boils. My grandmother looked at the leg and said, "Well, it's time to try the ground ivy." She picked some of the herb from her garden, placed it in a metal strainer, and held it above a pot of boiling water. After the leaves were thoroughly steamed, she applied them directly to the infection, placed some waxed paper over the leaves, and bandaged it all together. The infection was nearly gone by the following day.

Parts used: Aerial parts.

Actions: Anodyne, anticatarrhal, antidiabetic, antiphlogistic, antisclerotic, appetizer, cholagogue, diuretic, expectorant, hemostatic, stomachic, tonic, vulnerary.

Medicinal virtues: Ground ivy has long been used in Russia to help increase appetite, reduce coughing, and improve digestion. Ground ivy infusions are especially recommended for treating gastritis, colitis, and diarrhea, as well as for relieving infections of the kidneys, liver, gallbladder, and urinary bladder. When gallstones are present, ground ivy is said to not only relieve inflammation, but also to help small stones (1 to 2 mm in size) pass through. It has also been used to treat a wide variety of other diseases, including malaria, gout, goiter, and deafness. Russian herbalists use freshly crushed and steamed leaves (or a concentrated infusion of leaves) for treating joint inflammation and even bone fracture.

In dermatology, ground ivy infusions are taken internally to treat eczema, itching, neurodermatitis, vasculitis, sores, and wounds. An infusion of this plant is also valued by herbalists as a soothing eyewash and as a mouthwash to relieve gum pain. A vinegar infusion of ground ivy leaves, rubbed into the skin twice a day, is effective for treating skin scabs.

Habitat and collection: Ground ivy can be found primarily in sunny hedge banks and in waste areas. Harvest the herb in early May while most of the flowers are still fresh.

Preparation and dosage: To prepare an infusion, add 1 cup (250 ml) of boiling water to 1 teaspoon (5 g) of crushed herb. Steep for 15 to 20 minutes and strain. Take ¼ cup (60 ml) 4 times a day. Decoctions and tinctures should not be prepared at home.

Caution: **Ground ivy can be toxic when taken in large amounts. Do not exceed the recommended dosage of 1 cup per day and limit the course of treatment to 7 days.**

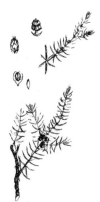

JUNIPER

Botanical name: *Juniperus communis.*
Family: Cupressaceae.

Juniper is easy to find; this evergreen plant stands out among many other plants that lose their leaves during the long Russian winters. Juniper also has a fresh, deodorizing aroma.

Russian czars and simple peasants alike used to decorate both their homes and their banyas with juniper boughs long before room deodorizers were invented. The juniper's distinctive aroma comes from its volatile chemical substances, which disinfect and improve air quality. Craftspeople always appreciated pale juniper wood for making their furniture and other objects. Juniper branches and needles were used to smoke fish and meats.

Parts used: Fruit.

Actions: Antiseptic, carminative, diuretic, expectorant, rubefacient, stimulant, stomachic, tonic.

Medicinal virtues: The main active substance of juniper is ether oil, which makes an excellent external antiseptic to treat diseases like cystitis. The oil easily penetrates the lungs, kidneys, liver, and urinary bladder and quickly acts to stimulate the body's mucous membranes. It is also used to stimulate digestion, relieve flatulence, and stimulate physiological or organic functioning in general. Juniper can be used as a diuretic. It is used to treat diseases of the kidney, bladder, and urinary tract, including kidney stones and urethritis.

Juniper berries are recommended as an expectorant for treating bronchitis. They can be eaten directly or brewed as a tea to treat symptoms of rheumatic joints, podagra, and arthritis by driving out mineral deposits and improving the exchange processes in the body's cells. These symptoms are also treated by rubbing juniper oil into the affected parts of the body to relieve pain. However, juniper is not recommended for treating nephritis and other acute inflammatory diseases.

Due to the precautions concerning treating kidney diseases with juniper preparations, juniper is usually prescribed for internal use for no more than two weeks at a time. Russian official medicine does not recommend it for pregnant women and discourages the use of prickly juniper *(Juniperus oxycedrus)* for treating any malady.

Habitat and collection: Juniper grows best in dry and rocky soil. Collect the berries in the autumn and dry them in a shady place.

Preparation and dosage: The most effective way to take juniper internally is to eat the fresh or dried berries. Begin by chewing 2 to 3 berries a day before breakfast and increase the number of berries on subsequent days until you are eating 15 a day. When that point is reached, decrease your intake by 1 berry daily for the next 10 days. At that point, you can stop taking them altogether.

To make a decoction, crush 10 berries, put them in 1 cup (250 ml) of hot water, and boil for 15 minutes. Cool for 45 minutes at room temperature and filter. Take 1 tablespoon (15 ml) 4 times a day before meals. A normal course of treatment lasts 2 weeks.

Caution: **Juniper preparations should not be taken by pregnant women or by individuals suffering from nephritis or other inflammatory diseases of the kidneys. Excessive doses of more than 45 to 50 berries at a time may cause poisoning.**

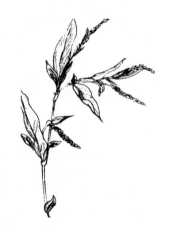

KNOTWEED
Botanical name: *Polygonum hydropiper.*
Family: Polygonaceae.
Also known as: Smartweed, water pepper.

The early Greeks and Romans made the earliest references to knotweed. Diascorides first mentioned its ability to clean wounds and reduce swelling. The famous scientist and alchemist Paracelsus described using knotweed as a rubefacient, while the sixteenth-century Italian botanist Mattiolus wrote about using the fresh juice of this herb on open sores on animals to repel attacking flies from the wounds. He also recommended placing this herb on fresh meat to protect it from insects. However, until the twentieth century herbals and other printed sources made no further mention of the herb.

After many years of relative obscurity among Russian herbalists, knotweed has recently been carefully researched and is now widely used in Russian official medicine. Scientific interest in knotweed was renewed in 1912 when the Russian pharmacist A. O. Piorovsky saw how folk herbalists used knotweed preparations to stop uterine and hemorrhoidal bleeding. He collected the herb and sent it to Dr. N. P. Kravlov, a professor of pharmacy at the Military Medicine Academy in St. Petersburg. Dr. Kravlov conducted extensive research, and confirmed the medicinal properties of knotweed. It is now part of the official herbal medicine tradition.

Parts used: Aerial parts.

Actions: Antiphlogistic, astringent, diaphoretic, diuretic, rubefacient.

Medicinal virtues: A commercially prepared liquid extract of knotweed is used to stop uterine bleeding and is available in Russia only with a doctor's prescription. Knotweed is also a major ingredient in commercially prepared hemorrhoidal treatments.

Russian folk herbalists use knotweed to gently stimulate blood circulation to the skin, and apply a compress of the fresh crushed herb on the back of the head to treat headache. Knotweed tea taken internally is recommended for treating hemorrhoids and as part of complex herbal remedies for stopping internal bleeding. Knotweed infusions are also used as a bath to reduce hemorrhoidal swelling. Some folk healers recommend using the infusion as a gargle for relieving toothache and for treating symptoms of laryngitis.

In many places, compresses made of fresh knotweed juice are applied to sores and wounds to help draw out pus. Shepherds and farmers use it on open skin sores on animals to prevent attacks from flies and other insects.

Habitat and collection: A ubiquitous plant, the hearty knotweed is found in waste places and fields in many parts of the world. It may be harvested from June through September after flowering. Collect the herb just before the stems begin to turn red, cutting the stems 4 to 8 inches from the ground.

Preparation and dosage: To make an infusion, add 1 cup (250 ml) of boiling water to 2 tablespoons (30 g) of herb. Steep for 5 minutes and filter. Take small sips of this infusion throughout the day.

Caution: Both internal and external preparations of this herb should be used only under the supervision of a physician or certified herbalist.

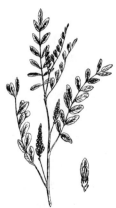

LADY'S MANTLE

Botanical name: *Alchemilla vulgaris.*
Family: Rosaceae.

Each leaf of this herb is rolled like a funnel, and in the morning a large drop of dew collects in the funnel and glistens like a pearl, taking on the colors of the rainbow in the morning sun. An old Russian folktale teaches children that gnomes never become old because they drink and wash their faces with morning dew from lady's mantle. In some parts of Russia, women rub their faces with the dew-covered leaves to remove skin blemishes.

Parts used: Aerial parts.

Actions: Astringent, depurative, diuretic, expectorant, stomachic, tonic, vulnerary.

Medicinal virtues: The Russian physicians M. A. and I. M. Nosal recommend drinking a lady's mantle decoction made with wine to treat lung and bronchial problems (including tuberculosis and bronchitis) as well as chronic diarrhea. An infusion of the herb made with water is popular in both official and folk medicine for treating a wide variety of health problems including stomach indigestion, intestinal gas, catarrh of the upper respiratory passages, tuberculosis, diabetes, dropsy, diseases of the liver and kidneys, and hernia.

When taken as a gargle, cold infusions of lady's mantle are useful in treating laryngitis. As a mouthwash, it helps heal mouth sores and ulcers. In dentistry, it is especially useful as a rinse after tooth extractions.

Infusions are also used to rinse nasal passages for those suffering from severe colds and nosebleeds. It is also recommended as a douche for women with excessive menstrual bleeding. Applied externally, an infusion of lady's mantle is a popular remedy for treating wounds, furuncles, and skin inflammations. In addition, some herbalists apply fresh leaves of the herb directly to boils.

Habitat and collection: Native to Europe, Asia, eastern Canada, and the northeastern part of the United States, lady's mantle is mostly found in damp places and shady wooded areas. The leaves and stems can be collected during July and August after the morning dew has dried.

Preparation and dosage: To make a wine decoction, boil 2 tablespoons (30 g) of the herb in 2 cups (500 ml) of white wine for 5 minutes.

For a water infusion, add 1 cup (250 ml) of boiling water to 1 tablespoon (15 g) of the herb. Steep for 15 minutes at room temperature. Filter. Drink ¹/₃ cup (80 ml) 3 times a day 10 minutes before meals. A course of treatment lasts 7 days.

To prepare a douche or skin poultice, pour 1¹/₂ quarts (1¹/₂ liters) of boiling water over 3 ounces (100 g) of herb. Allow to stand for 6 hours and strain. Use the rinse once a day for 3 to 5 days.

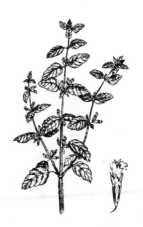

LEMON BALM
Botanical name: *Melissa officinalis.*
Family: Lamiaceae.
Also known as: Balm mint, bee balm,
    blue balm, cure-all, dropsy plant,
    garden balm, melissa, sweet balm.

One of the most popular herbs in Russia, lemon balm is highly valued for both culinary and medicinal use. Because it has a pleasant lemony taste, Russian cooks add fresh leaves to salads, use them to flavor both fish and chicken dishes, and add crushed, chopped leaves to stuffing and sauces. Dried leaves are also used in pillows for their pleasant smell.

Parts used: Aerial parts.

Actions: Antispasmodic, appetizer, calmative, carminative, diaphoretic, digestive, emmenagogue, stomachic.

Medicinal virtues: Because of its mild vasodilating properties, a lemon balm infusion can reduce the heart rate and lower blood pressure. In Russian official medicine, this quality is so well recognized that commercial preparations made from lemon balm are used to reduce blood pressure. Lemon balm contains a chemical called polyphenol that may help fight several strains of infection-causing bacteria. It also contains eugenol, an anesthetic that may help relieve wound pain. An infusion makes a good gargle to relieve inflammation of the gums and the mouth in general.

Lemon balm can stimulate the appetite and relieves vomiting and nausea as well as meteorism. It helps relieve gallbladder and kidney colic and calms spasms of the smooth muscles of the body, making it useful as an asthma preventive. Lemon balm fomentations are used externally to remove boils.

A tea (either hot or chilled) made from fresh flowers is enjoyed by Russians as a refreshing beverage. The tea is also used as a tonic to treat dizziness and as a detoxifier during pregnancy. It is used to alleviate painful, slow menstruation, while a lemon balm bath is recommended to promote the onset of menstruation. In addition, lemon balm tea is recommended for treating symptoms of insomnia, anemia, and gout, especially of the joints of the foot and the big toe. The tea is often prescribed to treat psychological problems like neurosis and depression. Herbalists are investigating the therapeutic effects of lemon balm tea to treat attention deficit disorder in children.

Habitat and collection: Lemon balm grows in almost any soil, but prefers moist areas along roadsides and in fields. It is also cultivated extensively throughout Europe and North America. Harvest the plant before or just after flowering. The fresh plant is more effective than the dried.

Preparation and dosage: As an infusion add 1 tablespoon (15 g) of fresh or dried herb or leaves alone to 1 cup (250 ml) of boiling water. Cover and steep for 5 to 10 minutes. Take ½ cup (125 ml) 3 times daily before meals or before bedtime.

To make an herbal bath, add 2½ cups (375 ml) of boiling water to approximately 10 ounces (300 g) of dried herb (or a handful of fresh herbs). Allow to steep for 10 minutes. Strain and pour into the bathtub.

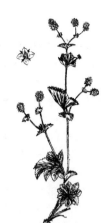

LICORICE

Botanical name: *Glycyrrhiza glabra.*

Family: Leguminosae.

Also known as: Licorice root, sweet licorice, sweet wood.

One of the most widely grown and appreciated herbs in the country, licorice is known in Russia as "sweet herb." It has been used since 5000 B.C.E. in all branches of world herbal traditions. Licorice root is comparable in importance to ginseng in the Chinese herbal tradition and is used in hundreds of recipes in ancient Chinese herbalogy.

In Russia, licorice is also highly valued for its use in confectionery. It is grown commercially in Russia and exported throughout the world. However, collection and selection of licorice for medicinal purposes requires far more care than for use in candy.

Parts used: Rootstocks.

Actions: Anodyne, antibacterial, antihistaminic, antiphlogistic, antispasmodic, diuretic, expectorant, laxative, mucilaginous, sudorific, tonic.

Medicinal virtues: Since licorice roots possess strong mucilaginous and expectorant qualities, they are used to treat inflammations of the upper respiratory tract like bronchitis, as well as acute respiratory diseases like chronic pneumonia. Licorice is also used in Russian herbal medicine to treat dyspepsia (shortness of breath and difficulty breathing) and throat diseases. It can also be used to treat stomach problems, such as inflammation of the mucous membrane of the stomach along with hyperacidity and peptic and duodenal ulcers.

In Russia, licorice root is a popular remedy for treating bladder and kidney ailments, gestational toxicosis (involving both excessive vomiting at the beginning of pregnancy and dropsy or edema at the end of pregnancy), and constipation.

A licorice root ointment is used in Russia to treat burns, eczema, lupus erythematosus, and hives. An infusion is used to treat cholelithiasis, chronic constipation, early stages of diabetes mellitus, and insignificant hypertonia.

The ability of licorice root infusions to neutralize poisons has been known in Russia since ancient times. It can neutralize the effects of chemical poisons, food poisoning, viruses, bacteria, and other toxins. Russian herbalists recommend giving licorice root tea with milk to children suffering from whooping cough and thrush.

In addition, licorice root possesses numerous biologically active elements that reduce blood cholesterol and aid in dissolving and removing cholesterol plaque in the blood vessels. It has a strong effect on the endocrine system and is reputed to have an overall tonic and stimulating effect on the entire body.

Habitat and collection: Licorice grows wild in southern Russia, Belarus, and Ukraine and is widely cultivated in other parts of the world. Harvest the rootstock from May to November.

Preparation and dosage: To prepare a decoction, add 1 tablespoon (15 g) of rootstocks to 2 cups (500 ml) of water. Bring to a boil, then simmer gently for 10 minutes. If necessary, add enough water to make two cups of the decoction. Allow to cool, then strain. Take $^1/_2$ cup (125 ml) 4 times a day after meals. Keep refrigerated.

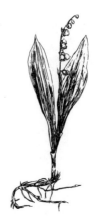

LILY OF THE VALLEY
Botanical name: *Convallaria majalis*.
Family: Liliaceae.

There are many Russian fairy tales about the lily of the valley. In one tale a young woman called the White Snow Maiden ran away from her wicked stepmother. As she ran, the necklace she wore fell apart. The fallen pieces became the lily of the valley.

In another tale, Volhva, the Water Queen, was in love with Sadko, a handsome musician. When she found out that he was deeply in love with a young girl who lived in a village near the river, she left the water to hear him play and sing to his beloved. When Volhva heard him play, bitter tears welled up in her beautiful blue eyes. They fell onto the ground and became the aromatic white flowers we know as lilies of the valley.

This herb has been known in Russian folk medicine since time immemorial. It was first introduced into official medicine by the noted surgeon F. I. Inozemtev in 1861.

Parts used: Aerial parts.

Actions: Antiseptic, cardiac, diuretic, emollient, laxative.

Medicinal virtues: Preparations made with this herb are effective for cardiac insufficiency. A Russian commercial preparation known as Corglickon is made from the leaves of this herb and is used to treat cardiac insufficiency and to calm the nervous system in general. An extract of the herb is also used to treat cardiac arrhythmia.

Lily of the valley is recommended for individuals who engage in very strenuous labor and for women during menstruation. Recent research has found that this herb contains antiphlogistic and vasodilator substances. The leaves in particular also contain high concentrations of vitamin C.

Folk healers have long used the herb to treat epilepsy and apoplexy. Some eye ailments are treated with a cold compress soaked in a liquid extract of this herb. It is also taken internally to relieve stomach pains and fever.

Habitat and collection: A popular garden plant, lily of the valley is found throughout the countryside in Europe (except in the extreme north and south), eastern Canada, and the northeastern United States. The plant flowers in May and June, when the leaves can be collected.

Preparation and dosage: To make a tincture for heart and nervous ailments, fill a 2-cup (500-ml), narrow-necked bottle three-quarters full with fresh herb. Pour 90-proof alcohol (such as vodka) into the bottle until it is full. Close and allow to stand for 2 weeks at room temperature. After 2 weeks, filter the liquid, which should be clear and light yellow in color. Add 10 to 15 drops to 1 cup of water and drink once a day after eating. Take for no longer than 3 to 5 days *under a doctor's supervision.*

Caution: Lily of the valley can be toxic in large doses. For this reason we recommend that this herb be taken only as directed by a qualified health-care professional.

LINDEN

Botanical names: *Tilia cordata,*
  Tilia europea.
Family: Tiliaceae.

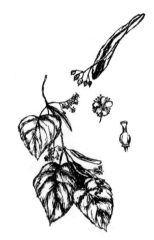

Linden is one of Russia's most popular trees. At least eleven different varieties of linden trees grow in the former Soviet Union, primarily in Russia, Belarus, and Ukraine. In some areas, the trees are cultivated for their medicinal properties. An estimated twenty-seven million acres are devoted to linden tree plantations.

When I was a child, we drank linden flower tea whenever we had a cold or a cough. Because of its pleasant taste and aroma, we also enjoyed it as a hot beverage. It does not need to be sweetened, although some people like to add a small amount of honey.

My mother would often take us to the country each spring to pick linden flowers. We would return home with large bags of fresh flowers, which we would lay out to dry. The flowers often lasted far into the next winter. When my mother didn't have time to take us into the country, she picked the flowers from trees on our street and put them in a plastic bag.

Parts used: Flowers.

Actions: Anticoagulant, cholagogue, disinfectant, expectorant, nervine, sudorific.

Medicinal virtues: Linden flower tea is a popular remedy for treating coughs and colds and is considered one of the best remedies for relieving symptoms of bronchitis and warding off influenza. It is also used to relieve kidney diseases and prevent children's infections. Linden tea is a strong and safe nervine and is widely used to relieve headaches, anxiety, and nervous tension.

Herbalists prescribe the tea as a gargle and mouthwash to relieve symptoms of tonsillitis and inflammations of the mouth. It is sometimes combined with baking soda and propolis.

Used externally, a strong infusion of unstrained tea can be applied to treat hemorrhoids, rheumatism, podagra, and burns. Some sources recommend using infusions of young linden leaves and buds for these purposes as well. Folk healers sometimes recommend using linden flower infusions cooled to room temperature as a face wash to improve the elasticity and fresh appearance of the skin.

Habitat and collection: Pick the flowers in the springtime when the tree is in full flower. Avoid collecting flowers from branches touched by leaf-eating worms. Dry the flowers in a well-ventilated, shady spot.

Preparation and dosage: To make an infusion, add 1 cup (250 ml) of boiling water to 1 tablespoon (15 g) of flowers. Steep for 10 minutes and then strain. Take 1 cup 3 times a day after meals. When cooled to room temperature, this tea can also be used externally twice daily.

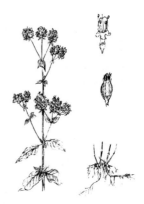

MARJORAM
Botanical name: *Origanum vulgare.*
Family: Labiatae.

Russian peasants have traditionally called marjoram "sweetly scented" because of its pleasant, aromatic smell. In times past, inhabitants of Russian farms and villages used to hang this herb in their homes as a natural deodorizer. Since modern commercial deodorizers are too expensive for many country people in Russia today, the marjoram plant still retains its early appeal.

Marjoram not only smells good but also has a calming effect on those who use it. Marjoram tea can provide restful sleep for those suffering from insomnia and is even believed to enhance dreams. There is an old folk song describing a Russian wife whose husband is going off to war. He tells her not to cry but to stuff her pillow with "sweetly scented" so that she would dream of him.

Parts used: Aerial parts.

Actions: Antiphlogistic, antispasmodic, calmative, carminative, diaphoretic, emmenagogue, expectorant, sedative, stomachic, tonic, vulnerary.

Medicinal virtues: Marjoram preparations have a calmative effect on the central nervous system, and official healers have used it to treat insomnia, nervous tension, and hypertension. It is also used to treat atherosclerosis. As a tonic, this herb is used to treat gastritis and to aid intestinal peristalsis. A marjoram infusion is used to treat constipation and excessive gas and to relieve symptoms of cold and flu.

As an expectorant, marjoram is used to treat diseases of the respiratory tract, including chronic and acute bronchitis. A strong marjoram tea can induce abundant perspiration. Taken internally, a marjoram infusion helps to relieve menstrual cramps, excessive sexual erethism, and amenorrhea. A mixture of marjoram, raspberry, and coltsfoot (see recipe in "The Respiratory System") makes a good remedy for the relief of colds, coughs, and whooping cough.

Externally, a marjoram infusion is used as a wash and bath for treating skin problems, including eczema, wounds, and skin inflammations. It can also be used as a gargle to relieve chronic tonsillitis and as a mouthwash to relieve gum diseases like gingivitis.

Marjoram enjoys even wider use among traditional folk healers in Russia. Marjoram infusions are used to treat headache, rheumatism, epilepsy, tuberculosis, wheezing cough, and rickets and scrofula in children. Marjoram compresses are applied externally on furuncles and abscesses. An oil made from this herb is often applied directly to an aching tooth and can be applied to the temples to relieve headache due to stress. Russian folk healers believe that using an infusion of marjoram regularly to wash the hair can retard hair loss.

In addition to its medicinal uses, fresh and dried marjoram is a popular seasoning for salads, vegetables, and egg dishes. In Russia, it is also traditionally added to meat, beans, and peas.

Habitat and collection: Wild marjoram is native to the Mediterranean region of Europe but is widely cultivated in North America. Harvest between July and September.

Preparation and dosage: To make an infusion, add 1 cup (250 ml) of boiling water to 1 tablespoon (15 g) of herb. Steep for 15 minutes. Strain and take 3 times a day a half hour before meals.

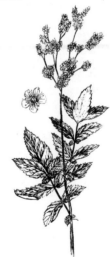

MEADOWSWEET

Botanical name: *Filipendula ulmaria.*
Family: Rosaceae.
Also known as: English meadowsweet,
    brideswort, queen of the meadow.

For centuries, meadowsweet has been appreciated throughout Europe for its beauty, aroma, and medicinal properties. The English herbalist John Gerard wrote that "the leaves and flowers of meadowsweet farre excell all other strowing herbs for to deck up houses . . . for the small thereof makes the heart merrie and joyful." Meadowsweet flowers are often scattered in the houses where wedding festivals took place, thus earning meadowsweet the nickname "brideswort."

Russian herbalists often tell the story of a brave knight named Kudryash, the strongest man in the village. One morning he woke up filled with fear of his impending death. He was so fearful that he carefully avoided any confrontations that could lead to a fight. However, during this time a band of marauding thieves were planning to raid the village, and the local people looked to Kudryash for leadership.

Ashamed of his fear and feeling powerless against the band of thieves, Kudryash could not sleep nights. One morning he went to the river to drown himself but came upon a beautiful girl instead. In her hand was a garland made of meadowsweet flowers, and she told him to wear it for protection.

Later that day he fearlessly led the villagers into battle, and they soundly defeated the invaders. Kudryash was declared the savior of the town and was celebrated for his courage and leadership by the populace.

Like willow, meadowsweet contains salicin, the primary ingredient found in aspirin. It has been researched throughout Europe, although the bulk of investigations have been carried out at the University of St. Petersburg. Salicylic acid has been found in meadowsweet flowers, along with heliotropin, vanillin aldehyde, and several other compounds used in commercial medications.

Parts used: Aerial parts, roots.

Actions: Anthelmintic, antibacterial, antiphlogistic, astringent, calmative, cholagogue, diaphoretic, diuretic, hemostatic, stomachic, tonic, vulnerary.

Medicinal virtues: Meadowsweet is used widely in both folk and official medical practice. A decoction made of the shredded root and flowers is recommended for nervous disorders, such as hysteria and neurosis as well as hypertension. It is also used as a diuretic to treat inflammatory disorders of the kidney and bladder, including cystopyelitis (cystitis with inflammation of the pelvis or the kidney) and difficulties with urination.

A decoction made from meadowsweet flowers and leaves helps reduce coughing and relieve bronchitis, bronchial asthma, and tonsillitis with nasal congestion, as well as influenza and the common cold.

An infusion of meadowsweet flowers is used to treat stomach and duodenal ulcers and can relieve symptoms of bacillary dysentery. It is also effective in treating podagra and rheumatism.

An infusion of meadowsweet leaves (or an ointment made from the leaves) is used externally to reduce inflammatory problems related to bones (such as arthritis) and has a strong curative effect on trophic sores, burns, old wounds, skin rash, boils, insect bites, purulent fistulas, and even smelly feet.

Habitat and collection: Meadowsweet can be found in deep meadows throughout northern Europe, the eastern United States, and southeastern Canada. Harvest when the flowers are in full bloom, usually between June and August. Dry at room temperature.

Preparation and dosage: To prepare a decoction, add 1 teaspoon (5 g) of root to 2 cups (500 ml) of hot water. Cover loosely and simmer for 30 minutes. Strain while still hot and add previously boiled water to achieve the original 2 cups. Take 1 tablespoon (15 ml) 3 times a day after meals. For a root decoction as a wash, add 1 tablespoon (15 g) of powdered roots to 1 quart (1 liter) of boiled water.

To make an infusion, add 1 teaspoon (5 g) of herb to 1 cup (250 ml) of hot water. Steep for 15 minutes and strain. Take 1 to 2 tablespoons (15 to 30 g) 3 times a day before meals.

To make an ointment, gradually mix 1 tablespoon (15 g) of well-crushed roots with 3 ounces (100 g) of petroleum jelly. Apply to affected areas once or twice a day.

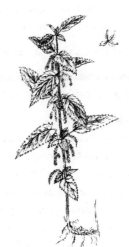

NETTLE
Botanical name: *Urtica dioica.*
Family: Urticaceae.
Also known as: Stinging nettle.

Nettle has long occupied an important place in both folk-herbal tradition and official Russian medical research. Mention of this herb can be found in medical texts dating from the seventeenth century. Although physicians at that time did not realize that bacteria can cause disease, they nonetheless were using a variety of bactericidal preparations from herbs such as nettle.

While nettle is widely recognized for its immune-enhancing properties today, during the seventeenth century physicians' primary interest in nettle centered around the treatment of wounds. One Russian herbal of that period, (known simply as *The Herbal Book*) describes the use of nettle: "We chew raw nettle, mash it and apply it to fresh wounds, and so we clean and heal the wounds." For old, infected wounds, the practitioner was advised to crush both the nettle leaves and seeds, and add salt: "Apply to old infected wounds and they will get the dead tissue out and heal the wounds." Three centuries later, medical science discovered bacteria, which offered a scientific explanation for the success of old herbal recipes like nettle and salt.

Parts used: Leaves.

Actions: Antiphlogistic, astringent, cardiac, carminative, cholagogue, depurative, digestive, diuretic, emmenagogue, expectorant, febrifuge, galactagogue, hemostatic, purgative, stomachic, tonic, vulnerary.

Medicinal virtues: An infusion made from nettle has long been used to treat all chronic diseases resulting from lowered immune function. Rich in iron and vitamin C, nettle has been prescribed for people suffering from anemia and vitamin deficiency. It is also taken for the relief of arthritis as well as rheumatism of the muscles and joints.

Russian herbalists recommend nettle preparations for treating diseases of the gastrointestinal tract, including diarrhea and constipation. It is also considered an effective remedy for treating acute and chronic inflammation of the small intestine as well as stomach colic, indigestion, and meteorism. Nettle infusions have also been found effective for relieving liver diseases, kidney, bladder, and gallbladder problems, urinary stones, nephritis, and cystitis. As a hemostatic, nettle infusions are recommended for treating renal, uterine, and intestinal hemorrhage and nasal bleeding.

Russian physicians have found that nettle helps tone the cardiovascular system and use it to treat atherosclerosis and to reduce cholesterol levels in blood. It has also been used successfully to treat malaria. Nettle is also recommended for treating bronchitis and is often part of complex herbal recipes for the treatment of tuberculosis.

Fresh nettle juice promotes the flow of milk in nursing mothers and helps normalize the menstrual cycle. Nettle leaves reduce blood sugar, so it is often recommended for patients suffering from diabetes.

In official dermatology, nettle infusions are recommended to treat vasculitis, furunculosis, acne, eczema, psoriasis, neurodermatitis, and vitiligo. Compresses of nettle (either as decoctions or infusions) help relieve burns and wounds.

In folk medicine, the entire herb is often used. A preparation made from nettle roots is used to relieve cough, while a juice made from leaves stops bleeding. Fresh leaves and roots may also be used for premature gray hair. An infusion of dry leaves is used on the scalp to treat dandruff and help stop hair loss. When taken internally, a nettle infusion is reputed to be helpful for relieving painful menstruation as well as other female problems. A decoction made from the whole herb may be used for headaches. The herb decoction, made with honey, improves the function of the heart, liver, and kidneys and relieves symptoms of gastritis and anemia. A root decoction is used to treat whooping cough, and a decoction of flowers relieves diabetes.

Habitat and collection: Nettle is a perennial herb found throughout the temperate regions of the world. A hearty plant, it grows wild along roadsides and in waste places. Collect the herb when it blossoms in June or July. Be sure to wear gloves to prevent getting "stung" by the nettles.

Preparation and dosage: To make an infusion, add 1 cup (250 ml) of boiling water to 1 tablespoon (15 g) of dried leaves. Steep for 10 minutes. Drink 1 cup (250 ml) 3 times a day.

To prepare nettle juice, wash the leaves well in cold water and rinse in hot boiled water. Process the leaves in a food grinder and dilute pulp by adding 3 parts of water for every 1 part of pulp. Boil the mixture gently for 3 to 5 minutes. Remove from heat, allow to cool, and strain. Take 1 to 2 tablespoons (15 to 30 ml) 3 times a day before meals. The juice can be refrigerated in a tightly closed container for up to a week.

To make a decoction, add 2 tablespoons (30 g) of dried leaves to 1 cup (250 ml) of water. Bring to a boil then simmer gently for 5 minutes, stirring from time to time. Cover and let stand for an hour. Strain. Drink ⅓ cup (80 ml) 3 times a day.

Caution: Do not drink more than 3 cups of nettle tea per day because the tea stimulates powerful inner cleansing.

Oak

Botanical names: *Quercus robur* (English oak),
    Quercus rubra (red oak),
    Quercus alba (white oak).
Family: Fagaceae.

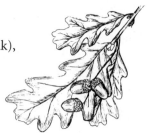

The oak tree has long been considered one of the world's most sacred trees. The ancient Greeks believed that the oak was the special tree of Zeus and that Zeus could be heard as rustling wind through the oak tree leaves at Dodona. The Druids worshipped oak trees and often performed their most important religious ceremonies in oak groves. The Lithuanians considered the oak sacred: There were no less than seventeen orders of priests devoted to worshiping the oak in that country before the fifteenth century. During religious ceremonies, offerings from the local people were often placed under the biggest trees to secure good health and abundant crops.

The oak also enjoys a long history as a healer and nurturer of humanity. Many native cultures depended on acorns for food and discovered its ability to stop bleeding and diarrhea, stimulate urination, and reduce fever. Russian folk healers have long prescribed spending time in oak forests. They believe that doing so is relaxing and promotes better sleep.

Part used: Bark.

Actions: Antiphlogistic, astringent, disinfectant, hemostatic, stomachic, styptic, vulnerary.

Medicinal virtues: Oak bark decoction possesses excellent astringent and hemostatic properties. It is prescribed by herbalists as a gargle for relieving inflammations of the throat, including hoarseness. As a mouthwash, it is considered an effective treatment for inflammations of the gums, including stomatitis, gingivitis, and bleeding gums.

Cold compresses made from oak bark decoctions are used externally to treat a variety of skin problems, including purulent sores, weeping eczema, burns, and bedsores. They also help to reduce swelling as a result of frostbite. In folk dermatology, oak bark baths are prescribed for treating symptoms of allergic dermatosis. They also reduce the predisposition of the feet and hands to excessive perspiration. In Russia, a commercially prepared ointment made from oak bark is used to heal extremely dry skin.

As a wash, an oak bark decoction is used to treat trichomoniasis, a parasitic infestation, as well as inflammation of the vagina and vaginal bleeding.

When used internally, oak bark decoctions are recommended for treating intestinal problems like diarrhea and dysentery. They are also considered effective for relieving chronic intestinal inflammations, as well as inflammation of the bladder and urinary tract.

Habitat and collection: There are many species of oak tree. Several hundred can be found in Russia alone. Oak grows in forests throughout Europe and North America.

Remove the young bark in thin patches from slender branches or the trunk. Take special care not to take the bark from the entire circumference of the trunk, which will kill the tree. Collect the bark in April or May.

Preparation and dosage: To make a decoction for internal use, place 1 teaspoon (5 g) of chopped bark into 1 cup (250 ml) of water. Bring to a boil, then reduce heat and simmer for 10 minutes, adding extra water from time to time to maintain the original water level. Strain. Drink 1 cup (250 ml) 3 times daily. This decoction may also be used as a styptic for burns and wounds.

To prepare a decoction for a healing bath or vaginal douche, use 2 tablespoons (30 g) of bark per 2 quarts (2 liters) of water. Bring to a boil and simmer for 10 minutes. Allow to cool and strain.

Caution: **Drinking more than the recommended amount may cause vomiting.**

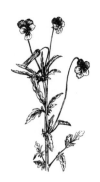

PANSY

Botanical name: *Viola tricolor.*
Family: Violaceae.
Also known as: Garden violet, heart's ease,
Johnny jump-up, stepmother.

The pansy has several different (and amusing) names in the Russian language. It is usually called "Anuta's eyes," because the petals appear to be the laughing eyes of a happy young lady. The pansy is also nicknamed "Ivan and Maria" after the two most popular male and female names in Russia. This name came about because the two darker, larger violet petals of the flower (Ivan) appear to embrace the three paler violet-yellow petals (Maria).

Although primarily known as a garden flower of outstanding beauty, this herb attracted the attention of Russian gardeners over a century ago. It is now cultivated throughout Russia in all colors, shapes, and varieties for both medicinal and ornamental purposes. It is among the most beautiful flowering herbs in the world.

Parts used: Aerial parts.

Actions: Antibacterial, calmative, carminative, demulcent, diuretic, expectorant, laxative, purgative, sudorific.

Medicinal virtues: An infusion of this herb is a good remedy for treating acute respiratory diseases like bronchitis and whooping cough. It also tends to reduce inflammation of the trachea (windpipe). Pansy is also useful for reducing inflammation of the urinary tract and is a common folk remedy for treating kidney stones. A pansy infusion is an effective remedy for treating inflammations in the gastrointestinal tract and is used to treat symptoms of dysentery. Russian herbalists also prescribe pansy infusions for treating atherosclerosis, arthritis, joint inflammations (especially rheumatism), gout, rickets in children, and as a preventive remedy for people who have previously suffered heart attacks.

Dentists prescribe a pansy gargle for inflammations of the mouth resulting from periodontal disease. Retaining a mouthful of pansy gargle for several minutes is often recommended for relieving toothache.

In folk medicine, pansy tea (in Russia, it is sold commercially under the name of Averin) is taken internally for cough. Pansy washes and compresses are widely used to treat a variety of skin diseases, including itching, eczema, psoriasis, allergic dermatitis, blackheads, and furunculosis.

Habitat and collection: The pansy species originated in the fields and meadows of Europe, but it is widely cultivated throughout North America. It prefers bright or slightly shady places in rich, woodland-type soil.

The plant is collected during flowering from May to August. Dry in a shady place. You can store this herb in a wooden or glass container for up to two years.

Preparation and dosage: To prepare an infusion, add 1 tablespoon (15 g) of the dried herb to 1 cup (250 ml) of boiling water. Cover and steep for 15 minutes. Strain. Take $^1/_3$ cup (80 ml) 3 to 4 times daily after meals.

Caution: **An overdose of this herb can cause nausea and vomiting, while excessive or prolonged use can cause skin problems.**

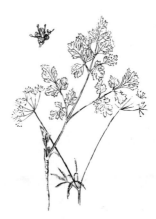

PARSLEY
Botanical name: *Petroselinum crispum.*
Family: Umbelliferae.

Parsley was first discovered by the ancient Greeks, who called it petro-selenium, meaning "growing on stones." At first, it was used primarily as an ornamental plant for decorating homes and for making garlands for the hair. An herbalist finally discovered the healing properties of this herb.

The Greeks brought parsley to Russia between the tenth and eleventh centuries. Petroselenium soon became a common houseplant, especially among people residing near the Black Sea. By the twelfth century, parsley was well known in other parts of Russia, as well as in the area that is today France, Holland, and Germany.

The Russian name *petrosila,* derived from petroselenium, means "Peter's strength." Although like the Greeks the Russians always valued parsley as an ornamental plant, they used it medicinally from the beginning. The herbal *Refreshing Windtown,* published in 1672, states that with petrosila herb "stones ran out of the bladder and kidneys, take out weakness of the liver, bellies sometimes make."

Parts used: Aerial parts, seeds.

Actions: Anesthetic, antiphlogistic, antiseptic, antispasmodic, appetizer, carminative, cholagogue, diaphoretic, disinfectant, diuretic, emmenagogue, stomachic.

Medicinal virtues: As a diuretic, parsley is used for treating kidney and cardiovascular diseases accompanied by edema. Both infusions and decoctions made from leaves and seeds are effective for treating symptoms of nephrolithiasis and inflammation of the mucosa of the urinary tract. Parsley fights bad breath, kills germs, and soothes gum inflammation and mucosa in the mouth.

Parsley is recommended for liver problems, stomach disorders, and urination disorders in children. It is also good for dyspepsia. It may be taken to help regulate menstruation (it stimulates the muscles of the uterus), uterine hemorrhage, and prostatitis.

A parsley decoction is effective for treating diseases of the blood vessels. It has a tonic effect on the veins and capillaries. It is also believed to slightly reduce blood sugar levels and is prescribed for diabetes.

Parsley is rich in vitamins and minerals (especially vitamin A, vitamin C, niacin, potassium, calcium, magnesium, and iron) and is recommended for people recovering from operations and who suffer from poor vision. It is also recommended to maintain good vision.

In dermatology, fresh parsley juice in combination with a root decoction and lemon juice is used to remove freckles and other forms of skin pigmentation. A root decoction is used by herbalists to prevent sunburn. Parsley is recommended for treating bruises, abscesses, allergic dermatitis, psoriasis, vasculitis, vitiligo, and other skin problems. It also helps treat mosquito bites, bee stings, and even snakebite. A highly concentrated decoction kills scalp vermin.

Habitat and collection: Parsley is primarily a garden herb. Collect the leaves during the growing season and the seeds in July.

Preparation and dosage: To make a cold infusion, take ¹/₂ teaspoon (2¹/₂ g) of seeds and add to 2 cups (500 ml) of water. Cover and allow to stand for 8 hours. Strain. Take 2 tablespoons (30 ml) 4 to 5 times daily.

To prepare a decoction, add 1 tablespoon (15 g) of any part or parts of the fresh herb to 2 cups (500 ml) of boiling water. Continue to boil for 30 minutes. Strain and add additional water so that you have the original 2 cups. Take 2 tablespoons (30 ml) 3 to 4 times a day before meals.

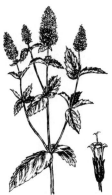

PEPPERMINT
Botanical name: *Mentha piperita.*
Family: Labiatae.

Peppermint is one of humanity's oldest and most loved herbs. As both a flavoring and a medicinal, it was cultivated by the ancient Egyptians for its volatile oil. The Greeks and Romans crowned themselves with peppermint at their feasts and used it in their wines and sauces. Although ancient manuscripts reveal that early Greek physicians used peppermint for healing, it was not introduced as a medicinal herb in Europe until the middle of the eighteenth century.

Like many others in Europe and the Americas, Russians are fond of peppermint and use it as a flavoring in sauces and wine and as a refreshing herbal tea taken either cold or hot. Its varied medicinal qualities also make peppermint a highly prized medicinal plant used by folk healers and official physicians alike.

Parts used: Aerial parts.

Actions: Anodyne, antibacterial, antiseptic, antispasmodic, appetizer, calmative, cardiac, carminative, cholagogue, expectorant, sedative, stomachic.

Medicinal virtues: Peppermint is used by Russian herbalists to treat a wide variety of stress-related disorders, including anxiety, hysteria, and insomnia. It has also been proven of value in alleviating symptoms of a number of heart-related problems like stenocardia and cardioneurosis. Herbalists use peppermint infusions to treat gallbladder inflammation, gallstones, and flatulence.

Peppermint tea makes an excellent appetizer. It improves digestion and reduces vomiting due to nervousness. Infusions are used to alleviate gastric spasms and colic, gastric hypoacidity, nausea, and vomiting, as well as halitosis (bad breath) due to dyspepsia. They are also recommended for treating respiratory tract inflammations as well as migraine headaches. Peppermint is also a popular remedy for cold and flu sufferers. Russian women take it regularly to relieve painful or scanty menstrual periods.

Russians use an infusion of peppermint as a gargle to treat mouth inflammation and toothache and apply diluted peppermint oil directly on hemorrhoids to relieve pain and swelling. In dermatology, peppermint compresses are applied on the skin for eczema and psoriasis, and ground fresh leaves are placed on the skin to relieve fungal infections.

Habitat and collection: Peppermint is widely cultivated throughout Europe and North America. However, it has been known to "escape" from gardens and can often be found growing along the banks of streams and in wastelands. Harvest the herb just before flowering, usually in July.

Preparation and dosage: To prepare an infusion, add 1 heaping teaspoon (7 g) of leaves or stems to 1 cup (250 ml) of boiling water. Cover and steep for 5 to 10 minutes. Take ½ cup (125 ml) twice a day before lunch and dinner.

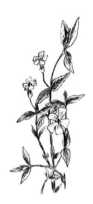

PERIWINKLE
Botanical name: *Vinca major, Vinca minor.*
Family: Apocynaceae.

Periwinkle is one of the most studied herbs in Russia. Used by humans for thousands of years, periwinkle is mentioned in both ancient Chinese and Greek herbals for treating high blood pressure. Folk healers from the south Caucasus mountains (in what is now Georgia and Armenia) used periwinkle to heal war wounds. It was also widely used for relieving symptoms as varied as toothache and diarrhea. After being discovered by official medicine more than sixty years ago, scientists have been able to isolate more than 117 types of alkaloids from this herb.

Parts used: Aerial parts.

Actions: Antiphlogistic, astringent, depurative, sedative, vasodilator, vulnerary.

Medicinal virtues: A periwinkle decoction is often prescribed by Russian herbalists for treating hypertension. However, periwinkle is better known in Russian herbalism for its astringent properties, especially in reducing excessive menstrual flow and in curbing blood loss between periods. As an astringent, it is also helpful in treating nasal bleeding and diarrhea. A periwinkle decoction is used externally to treat minor wounds, while a periwinkle infusion, used externally, is an effective treatment for skin rash and itching. Drinking periwinkle tea has a calming effect on the central nervous system and is recommended for people who are nervous and tense. In Russia, official and folk herbalists prescribe a periwinkle gargle for relieving inflammation of the mouth and symptoms of pharyngitis; you can also simply chew the herb for this purpose as well.

Habitat and collection: Periwinkle grows wild throughout northern Europe, but is a popular addition to both European and American herb gardens. Collect the herb in late spring after flowering.

Preparation and dosage: To make a decoction, take 1 teaspoon (5 g) of dry, well-crushed leaves and add to 1 cup (250 ml) of water. Heat to boiling, then reduce heat and simmer for 15 minutes. Cool for 1 hour and strain. Take 1 to 2 tablespoons (15 to 30 ml) every 2 hours.

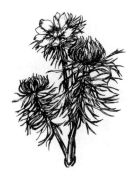

PHEASANT'S EYE
Botanical name: *Adonis vernalis.*
Family: Ranunculaceae.
Also known as: False hellebore, oxeye,
    sweet vernal.

In Russia, this old and important folk remedy is known as "burning flower" because of its bright and colorful appearance as it blooms profusely throughout the Russian steppes. Botanical sources dating from the seventeenth and eighteenth centuries indicate that the herb and its roots were widely used for treating a variety of heart and kidney diseases. It was also a popular neuralgia cure during the 1800s. From 1876 through 1879, Dr. N. A. Bubnov, a Russian physician who practiced in the Varonez area, learned much about this herb from local folk herbalists. He collected the herb and began researching it under the guidance of Dr. S. P. Botkin, one of Russia's most famous medical scientists. Since Bubnov's time, pheasant's eye preparations have been widely used in official medicine for treating a variety of cardiac problems, including coronary insufficiency.

Parts used: Aerial parts.

Actions: Antispasmodic, calmative, cardiac, diuretic.

Medicinal virtues: Like periwinkle, a source of digitalis, pheasant's eye is a cardioactive glycoside. This means that it can help normalize excessive contractions of the heart as well as irregular heartbeat. It also has been found to have a calming effect on the central nervous system. As a diuretic, pheasant's eye helps reduce liver enlargement and reduces edema in general. Russian folk herbalists use pheasant's eye preparations to help reduce kidney inflammation and to treat a variety of infectious diseases, including influenza and scarlet fever. They also report that pheasant's eye is effective for relieving shortness of breath.

Habitat and collection: Pheasant's eye grows wild in central Europe and is often found near corn fields. It is cultivated as well. Cut the herb 4 to 6 inches (10 to 15 cm) above the ground.

Preparation and dosage: To make a decoction, place 4 teaspoons (20 g) of crushed herb in a pot and add 2 cups (500 ml) of water. Heat to a boil, then reduce heat and simmer for 5 minutes. Steep at room temperature for 30 minutes. Strain. Take 1 tablespoon (15 g) 5 to 6 times a day.

Caution: **Pheasant's eye can be toxic if taken improperly, and preparations made with this herb may cause adverse side effects among individuals suffering from stomach or duodenal ulcers, gastritis, or stenocardia. The use of cardiac remedies by those who are clinically untrained can be dangerous. For this reason, use this herb only after consulting with a qualified healthcare professional.**

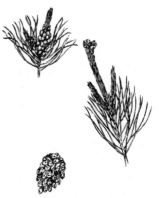

PINE

Botanical name: *Pinus strobus.*
Family: Pinaceae.

Pine is one of the most common trees growing in Russia, and at least thirty-three species of pine have proven medicinal properties. It can be found throughout the country and is the subject of many Russian songs and stories. Because pine trees are evergreens and never lose their needles despite heat, cold, storms, and drought, they are often regarded as trees of longevity and everlasting life. Pine trees impart a refreshing, pleasant scent and are believed to cleanse the lungs. This may be the reason why many of the earliest tuberculosis sanitariums in Russia were constructed in the middle of pine forests. In eastern North America, the most common pine species is the white pine *(Pinus strobus)* and was first used by Native Americans (including the Potawatomi, Objibway, and Tadoussac) for medicinal purposes.

Parts used: Buds, needles, resin from the inner bark.

Actions: Anodyne, anti-irritant, antiphlogistic, disinfectant, diuretic, expectorant.

Medicinal virtues: Pine buds are used as a decoction to treat coughs, inflammation of the respiratory tract, and infections due to colds, as well as bronchitis, rheumatism, and skin diseases. In Russia, boiling pine needles and inhaling the steam has long been valued for curing headache and relieving inflammation of the respiratory tract. In Russia, an infusion made from pine needles is said to be an excellent source of vitamin C, especially in winter. It is used in Russia as a prophylaxis against deficiency diseases such as scurvy.

Both pine needle infusions and extracts are used in bath water for their regulating effect on the central nervous system and in promoting healthy skin. In folk medicine, pine resin is used externally to heal chapped lips and nipples, as well as for treating furuncles and festering surface wounds.

Habitat and collection: *Pinus strobus* (known as eastern white pine) grows throughout Russia, and white pine can be found from western Canada to the eastern United States. Collect the cones in late summer; the leaves and bark can be harvested at any time.

Preparation and dosage: To make an infusion, add 1 teaspoon (5 g) of fresh chopped needles to 1 cup (250 ml) of boiling water. Steep for 10 minutes and strain. Let cool for 10 minutes. Drink 1 cup (250 ml) slowly 3 times a day.

To prepare as an inhalant, bring 6 tablespoons (90 g) of chopped pine twigs and needles to a boil in 2 quarts (2 liters) of water, and simmer gently for about 5 minutes. Place a towel over your head and inhale the steam for 10 to 15 minutes.

To prepare a pine bath, steep 6 tablespoons (90 g) of chopped pine twigs and needles in 3 pints (1¹/₂ liters) of water for 1 hour. Bring to a boil, then reduce heat and simmer for 5 minutes. Strain. Add the liquid to a bathtub filled with warm water. Soak in this water for 15 to 20 minutes.

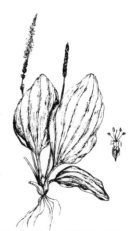

COMMON PLANTAIN

Botanical name: *Plantago major.*
Family: Plantaginaceae.
Also known as: Broad-leafed plantain,
    greater plantain, waybread, white man's foot.

Common plantain used to be considered a weed in both the United States and Russia. In Russia today, however, it is so highly regarded that it is specially cultivated for pharmaceutical use.

Centuries ago, plantain was especially prized by travelers in Russia. Travel then, unlike today, was undertaken only under great necessity, such as to flee persecution, find better cropland, or seek a better life. Before trains, trips of even a hundred miles in Russia were considered extremely difficult and often dangerous, with many travelers falling ill and dying en route. The serfs believed that this healing herb was a gift from God to travelers, and many would pray while spreading plantain seeds along the roadsides to help future travelers. Since the plantain seeds tended to stick to clothing and shoes, the plant was also propagated inadvertently by travelers. It is believed that this is how plantain was introduced to North America.

Parts used: Flowers, leaves, roots, seeds.

Actions: Antiphlogistic, antispasmodic, aperient, disinfectant, expectorant, hemostatic.

Medicinal virtues: It is no surprise why plantain was so appreciated by travelers. Fresh juice made of pounded and crumpled leaves and placed on the skin as a compress can be used to treat cuts, burns, wounds, and skin ulcers, as well as bee and wasp stings. Plantain leaves have also been used to treat snakebite; the most effective remedy is to pound and crush the leaves and apply them in a thick compress directly to the bite. The leaves draw off the poison, calm pain, and prevent swelling. Country people still use this old method when emergency medical treatment is not immediately available.

An infusion of plantain taken internally relieves headache and is a good expectorant for people suffering from bronchitis. It may also be used as a gargle to treat toothache.

The juice of fresh plantain leaves is prescribed by official Russian medicine to treat chronic gastritis, stomach ulcers, and ulcers of the duodenum with low and normal acidity. Plantain juice also is used to relieve stomach pain, improve appetite, and increase the acidity of the gastric juices. In 1965 a special over-the-counter preparation (known as Plantaglutcid) was formulated in Russia to treat stomach problems and sold throughout the country.

Powdered plantain seeds have been found to have a purgative effect. They are prescribed for diarrhea, which can occur as a side effect of tuberculosis.

Habitat and collection: Plantain is found throughout Russia and North America and grows wild in meadows, vacant lots, and on roadsides. The plant flowers from May to September.

Preparation and dosage: To make fresh plantain juice, cut the leaves, wash well in cold water, and then dip into boiling water for a few seconds. Blend the leaves in a food grinder or processor. Filter and squeeze well. If the juice turns viscous and thick in hot weather, dilute it with the same volume of water. Boil the juice for 1 to 2 minutes. Take 1 teaspoon (5 ml) 4 times a day, 15 to 20 minutes before mealtimes. The juice can also be dissolved in milk or soup.

To prepare an infusion, add 1 tablespoon (15 g) of herb to 1 cup (250 ml) of water. Let stand for 15 minutes. Take 1 tablespoon (15 g) 3 to 4 times a day before mealtimes. To make an infusion of plantain seeds, take 1 teaspoon (5 g) of powdered seeds and add to 1/2 cup (125 ml) of boiling water. Let cool for 10 minutes and take 1 teaspoon (5 g) (with the seeds) 2 to 3 times daily.

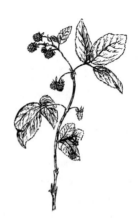

RASPBERRY

Botanical name: *Rubus strigosus.*
Family: Rosaceae.

Raspberry is perhaps one of nature's most generous gifts to humanity. Growing wild in forests and fields, it is also widely cultivated in gardens throughout Europe and North America.

Russians adore raspberries. Many either collect them in the forest every summer or grow them in their gardens. Russians use raspberries in a multitude of recipes, including wines, jams, and jellies. During the winter months, raspberry preserves serve as a primary remedy for treating colds and flu as well as for relieving high fevers. Russian children sometimes feign symptoms of illness in order to get a spoonful of delicious raspberry jelly from their parents.

Raspberry is mentioned in numerous Russian songs and poems as a sign of something sweet, attractive, and useful and as a symbol of the traditional Russian lifestyle so often cited in stories about Russian folkways.

Parts used: Flowers, fruit, leaves, roots.

Actions: Anodyne, antibacterial, antiemetic, antiphlogistic, antipyretic, antisclerotic, appetizer, astringent, diaphoretic, diuretic, hemostatic, refrigerant, stimulant, stomachic, tonic, vulnerary.

Medicinal virtues: A tea made of raspberries is recommended for treating symptoms of cold and flu and is an excellent refrigerant. It is also used as an addition to herbal antibacterial preparations to treat lung inflammations. Raspberries accelerate the process of recovery in cases of diseases of the gastrointestinal tract when accompanied by inflammation, vomiting, pain, and bleeding. The fresh fruit helps reduce blood sugar levels and is often recommended for treatment of diabetes. Raspberries also are recommended for treating sclerosis. In folk medicine, raspberries are prescribed for treating a wide variety of ailments, including diarrhea, anemia, chronic rheumatism, measles, and eczema. They are even prescribed to help make intoxicated people sober.

Folk herbalists prescribe a decoction made from raspberry tops with leaves to relieve symptoms of colds and flu, acute respiratory inflammation, and skin erysipelas. A leaf decoction is also good for relieving coughs, quinsy, tonsillitis, and high fever. A root decoction serves the same purpose and is considered effective for treating symptoms of diarrhea and colic as well. Root decoctions are also used to treat neuritis, neurasthenia, and bronchial asthma. A decoction made from roots and flowers is used by folk healers to treat leukorrhea in women.

Fresh leaves have a vulnerary effect and are considered useful for treating acne. Folk healers also recommend infusions of fresh leaves for treating diarrhea, inflammation of the stomach, the intestines, the lungs, and the mouth and throat.

Russian dermatologists use fresh raspberry juice (as well as a decoction made from dried fruits) taken internally to relieve hyperkeratosis, psoriasis, vitiligo, baldness, and purulent diseases of the skin. A decoction made from raspberry leaves and flowers is also used to treat food prurigo and hyperkeratosis. Used externally, raspberry juice is prescribed for treating acne, seborrhea, vitiligo, baldness, and premature graying of the hair.

Habitat and collection: Raspberry grows wild in many parts of Europe and North America. It is also widely cultivated. Harvest the leaves during the growing season, and collect the fruits whenever they are ripe.

Preparation and dosage: To prepare an infusion, add 2 tablespoons (30 g) of leaves to 1 cup (250 ml) of hot water. Allow to steep for 5 to 10 minutes. Take 2 to 3 cups (500 to 750 ml) every 1 to 2 hours as a traditional cold cure. You can also use this infusion as a gargle for the mouth and throat. A cold infusion is useful for treating diarrhea.

To make a decoction, add 1½ tablespoons (22 g) of roots to 1 cup (250 ml) of water. Heat to boiling and simmer gently for 30 to 40 minutes. Add additional hot water from time to time to maintain a constant level. Take ⅓ cup (80 ml) 3 to 6 times daily.

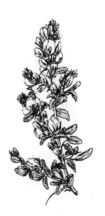

RESTHARROW
Botanical name: *Ononis spinosa.*
Family: Leguminosae.
Also known as: Cammock.

Russians sometimes call herbs with the Latin name *Ononis* "asses' herbs," because donkeys always liked to eat them while other animals avoided them, perhaps because of their unpleasant smell. However, in Russia restharrow has a more unusual history, primarily because its extract was used to harden metal into a steel known as *bulat.* It seems that the metalsmith's apprentice would dip the finished weapon in a vat containing a special liquid (of which restharrow extract was a part) and gallop away holding the sword aloft so that it would dry and harden in the wind. The sword would later be tested by striking it against an iron shield. Although scientists tried to discover the special metal-hardening property of restharrow, they were unsuccessful. However, official Russian medicine has investigated the medicinal properties of restharrow extensively and has confirmed many of its healing benefits.

Parts used: Roots.

Actions: Anodyne, antiphlogistic, aperient, coagulant, diuretic.

Medicinal virtues: Restharrow is helpful in treating urinary and kidney problems such as urinary catarrh, kidney inflammation, and rheumatism. It is recommended for people who tend to accumulate uric acid and are susceptible to kidney stones. As a diuretic, restharrow is effective without producing negative side effects. A decoction of restharrow has long been used by folk healers to treat eczema and other skin problems.

Recent medical research has found that this herb has a beneficial effect when used to treat hemorrhoids, chronic constipation, and infections of the anus. Infusions and decoctions of the roots are taken internally and are found to improve bowel movements, lower blood pressure, and reduce hemorrhoidal pain and swelling. For these problems, the average course of treatment lasts six weeks.

Habitat and collection: Restharrow is found in dry meadows and pastures throughout Europe, although it is often grown as a garden plant in North America.

Preparation and dosage: To make an infusion, add 1 tablespoon (15 g) of pounded roots to ½ quart (½ liter) of boiling water. Steep for 10 minutes, stirring occasionally. Filter. Drink ⅓ cup (80 ml) three times daily.

A decoction is made by adding 1 tablespoon (15 g) of pounded roots to 2 cups (500 ml) of boiling water. Reduce heat and simmer for 30 minutes. Filter and squeeze out additional moisture. Take ⅓ cup (80 ml) 3 times daily before mealtimes. The decoction can be stored in a refrigerator for a maximum of 2 days.

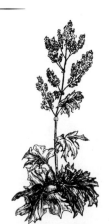
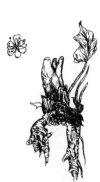

RHUBARB
Botanical name: *Rheum palmatum*.
Family: Polygonaceae.
Also known as: Turkey rhubarb,
   China rhubarb.

Rhubarb has an interesting history in Russia. Although the Swedish botanist K. Linney first described this herb, he had originally received rhubarb seeds from the Russian physician D. Groter in 1750.

First imported from China centuries before, rhubarb had been subject to a state monopoly on sales decreed by Czar Peter the Great in 1704. In 1736 the government began supervising its growth in special farms and soon began exporting rhubarb to western Europe. However, in an expedition between 1871 and 1873, the Russian explorer and scientist N. M. Przevalsky found rhubarb growing naturally in southern Russia, and several varieties of seeds collected by him were later grown at the State Botanical Garden in St. Petersburg. By the beginning of the nineteenth century, rhubarb was cultivated on large farms as an important medicinal herb.

Part used: Rootstocks.

Actions: Appetizer, astringent, cholagogue, purgative, tonic.

Medicinal virtues: In both official and folk medicine, rhubarb is often prescribed in combination with gentian and sweet flag. As a mild purgative, rhubarb is used to treat indigestion and diarrhea among both young children and elderly adults. As a cholagogue, it is recommended for treating liver problems, while its tonic properties make rhubarb infusions a popular remedy for relieving stomach and intestinal distress. In Russia, rhubarb is a popular ingredient in jam, candy, sauces, and cake fillings.

Habitat and collection: This plant is widely cultivated. The roots are harvested in October.

Preparation and dosage: To prepare a decoction, add 1 teaspoon (5 g) of dried rootstocks to 1 cup (250 ml) of water. Bring to a boil then simmer over low heat for 10 minutes. Strain. Drink this mixture twice a day, preferably after breakfast and dinner.

To make an alcohol infusion of rhubarb roots, gentian, and sweet flag, take equal proportions and add 1 part herbs to 10 parts 70-proof alcohol. It will be a transparent red or reddish-brown liquid with a flavorful, yet bitter taste. Take $^{1}/_{2}$ to 1 teaspoon ($2^{1}/_{2}$ to 5 g) 2 times a day before meals for constipation.

Caution: **Pregnant and nursing women should avoid taking rhubarb preparations. In addition, rhubarb may also turn the urine red, though this is not necessarily a negative sign.**

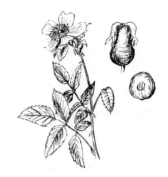

Rose Hips
Botanical name: *Rosa canina*.
Family: Rosaceae.
Also known as: Briar hip, dog rose,
    hip tree, briar rose.

Rose hips come from a species of wild rose, known as "dog rose," which is native to much of Europe, including Russia and Britain. The canine reference is attributed to the plant's daggerlike thorns, which later became known as "dag" and then "dog" in English.

In medieval times, the fruit of this flower was highly esteemed for its pleasant acidic taste. It was used to make preserves and sauces in Germany, while the Russians fermented the hips and made them into wine. According to Margaret Grieve's *A Modern Herbal,* one European writer observed centuries ago that: "Children with great delight eat the berries thereof when they are ripe and make chains and other pretty gewgaws of the fruit; cookes and gentlewomen make tarts and suchlike dishes for pleasure."

Parts used: Branches, fruit (hips), roots.

Actions: Astringent, cholagogue, digestive, diuretic, hepatic, tonic, vasodilator.

Medicinal virtues: As in North America, rose hips infusions are enjoyed in Russia primarily as a delicious tea that is rich in vitamin C. In addition to being used by herbalists to treat vitamin C deficiency, rose hips tea is also recommended as a cholagogue to treat liver diseases, including hepatitis. Russians also enjoy rose hips tea to prevent colds and other infectious diseases.

In folk medicine, decoctions of rose hips are prescribed (usually in addition to other herbal treatments) for their beneficial effects among people suffering from liver and kidney diseases, bladder inflammation, and heart problems. Because *Rosa canina* is a vasodilator, a decoction of hips is prescribed for people suffering from high blood pressure. It also relieves headaches and hyperacidity. A root decoction is prescribed to reduce blood pressure as well. Folk healers recommend a decoction made from branches to treat symptoms of dysentery, rheumatism, and radiculitis, which involves inflammation of the spinal nerve roots. Root decoctions are also prescribed for those with a tendency toward kidney or bladder stones.

Habitat and collection: The dog rose grows in fields and thickets and wherever hedges can be found. The plant blooms in midsummer, but gather the hips toward the end of September. Gather only the young branches.

Preparation and dosage: To make an infusion, add 1 teaspoon (5 g) of hips to 1 cup (250 ml) of hot water. Cover and steep for 5 to 10 minutes. Drink 1 cup (250 ml) 3 times a day as desired.

To prepare a decoction, add 3 tablespoons (45 g) of hips, fresh, young branches, or roots to 2 cups (500 ml) of boiling water. Continue to boil for 10 minutes, then steep for 8 hours. Strain. Take 1/2 cup (125 ml) 3 times a day.

ROWAN

Botanical name: *Sorbus aucuparia.*
Family: Rosaceae.
Also known as: European mountain ash,
  sorb apple.

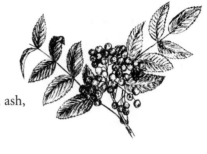

Rowan is one of Europe's most sacred trees. It played a major role in religious ceremonies of the Celts and the Druids and was reputed to protect people from evil spirits, believed at that time to be the primary cause of illness. In northern Europe, there are sayings such as, "No witch dare pass where rowans grow." In Russia, people used to grow rowan trees near the house to protect it against witches, warlocks, and ghosts. A cross made of rowan wood was often carried three times around houses, barns, or stalls to protect the inhabitants (whether human beings or farm animals) from evil. Smaller crosses were hung around the necks of farm animals to ward off disease and accidents.

Parts used: Flowers, fruit, leaves.

Actions: Antibacterial, antilithic, aperient, astringent, cholagogue, diuretic, hemostatic, purgative, tonic, vulnerary.

Medicinal virtues: Rowan is widely used in both folk and official healing traditions. As a popular tonic, it is widely used for health maintenance and disease prevention. In official medicine, a juice made from fresh rowanberries is used to treat gastritis and hypertension. A decoction made from rowanberries is recommended for bladder diseases, problems involving the bile ducts, kidney stones, and gallstones. It also reduces pain from rheumatism.

Because it is rich in beta carotene, vitamin C, and other essential nutrients, rowan tea is often recommended in cases of vitamin deficiency, anemia, and emaciation. It is also a good prophylactic for people suffering from atherosclerosis and is reputed to strengthen the veins and capillaries.

In folk medicine, a decoction of rowan flowers is prescribed for treating liver problems. It reduces the quantity of fats in the liver, thus stimulating liver metabolism. It also is used to reduce coughing and prevents goiter in women. A decoction made with vodka is often prescribed to treat hemorrhoids.

Rowanberries eaten fresh, as a juice, or in a jam are believed to reduce cholesterol in the blood and are viewed as a preventive for heart disease.

Fresh rowan leaves are applied to the skin to treat fungal infections, as well as a number of skin allergies.

Habitat and collection: Rowan is a deciduous tree that grows wild in the forests of Europe and western Asia. It is also a popular ornamental grown for both its beauty and its fruit. Collect the flowers in June and the berries in the fall.

Preparation and dosage: To make a rowan infusion, add 1 teaspoon (5 g) of fresh or dried berries to 1 cup (250 ml) of water. Bring to a boil, then let cool and strain. Take ¹/₃ cup (80 ml) 1 to 3 times a day.

To treat hypertension, take 1 tablespoon (15 ml) of juice 3 to 4 times a day before meals. To relieve gastritis, take 1 teaspoon (5 ml) of juice 20 to 30 minutes before meals.

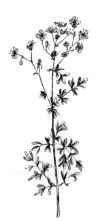

RUE

Botanical name: *Ruta graveolens.*
Family: Rutaceae.

Rue has long been appreciated for its healing powers. The Latin name *ruta* comes from the Greek *reuo* meaning "to set free," because the plant was able to heal people from many diseases. Hippocrates used rue as part of an antipoison remedy. In Europe during the Middle Ages, rue was said to possess magical powers against witchcraft and evil spells, which were often believed to cause illness. It was also known as the "herb of grace" because holy water was sprinkled from brushes made of rue at church ceremonies preceding Sunday's high mass.

Parts used: Flowers, leaves.

Actions: Anesthetic, antibacterial, anthelmintic, antiphlogistic, antispasmodic, appetizer, calmative, cardiac, carminative, emmenagogue, rubefacient, sedative, stimulant, stomachic, tonic, vulnerary.

Medicinal virtues: Official Russian herbalists use rue infusions primarily to treat disorders of the nervous system, including nervous spasms, heart spasms, spasms of the stomach and the intestinal muscles, and quickened palpitations of the heart (tachycardia). Rue is also used to relieve giddiness and breathing difficulties. Rue infusions promote the onset of menstruation, and herbalists often prescribe them for women whose periods are late.

Infusions made from rue leaves and used as a wash are recommended for treating a variety of skin problems, including skin rash, itchy scabs, bruises and sores; as an eyewash it can relieve suppurative eye inflammation.

In folk medicine, an infusion of rue leaves (which are collected during flowering) is recommended for people suffering from kidney stones. The herb decoction is used for treating disorders of the nervous system, as well as diarrhea, fever, and excessive menstrual bleeding. Rue infusions increase the appetite and aid digestion. They are also taken to expel intestinal worms.

In Russia, herbalists use rue infusions to treat chronic inflammation of the mouth, throat, and gastrointestinal tract, as well as stomach colic and inflammation of the stomach mucosa accompanied by gastric hypoacidity. They are also prescribed for bronchitis, pneumonia, and for people suffering from nervous tension and headaches.

Habitat and collection: Rue is native to southern Europe and northern Africa, but is widely cultivated in gardens throughout Europe and North America. Collect the herb in early summer before flowering. Dry in a shady place.

Preparation and dosage: To prepare an infusion, add 1 cup (250 ml) of boiling water to 1 tablespoon (15 g) of the herb. Steep for 10 to 15 minutes and filter. Take 3 times a day after meals.

To make a decoction, add 1 teaspoon (5 g) of dried herb to 2 cups (500 ml) of boiling water. Boil for 3 to 5 minutes. Allow to cool to room temperature and strain. Take $^1/_3$ to $^1/_2$ cup (83 to 125 ml) 3 times a day after meals.

Caution: **Excessive doses and prolonged use of rue preparations can cause mild poisoning. Since rue oil can bring about miscarriage, rue should not be used by pregnant women.**

RUPTUREWORT
Botanical name: *Herniaria glabra.*
Family: Caryophyllaceae.

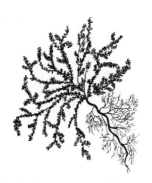

When I was twenty years old, I spent two months in a remote village in Belarus and was fortunate to stay with an old woman who practiced herbal medicine. One day I saw her hanging rows of a strange aromatic herb from the eaves of a shed behind her house. Eager to answer my questions, she told me that she was going to use the herb instead of soap, since commercially made soap was too expensive for her to buy in the store. Leading me to a pot of boiling water, the woman placed several handfuls of the herb in the pot, which soon produced a thick layer of foam. At first, I thought that she was having some fun at my expense, since I couldn't believe that you could make soap simply by placing an herb in boiling water. It was only later that she told me that while rupturewort could indeed be used as a soap, it also had numerous healing properties, which included the relief of ruptures or hernias.

Centuries ago, this herb attracted attention because rupturewort's rich lather washes out dirt from wool. At the present time, this herb has been researched so thoroughly in Russia and the rest of Eastern Europe (including the Czech Republic, Slovakia, Hungary, and Poland) that it is considered part of official medicine.

Parts used: Aerial parts.

Actions: Analgesic, diuretic.

Medicinal virtues: Since the advent of modern surgical methods, the use of rupturewort compresses has declined in the treatment of ruptured hernias. However, in folk medicine the herb is considered a specific remedy for acute inflammatory conditions as well as spasms in the bladder. When prepared as a tea, rupturewort is used to treat kidney problems and diseases of the urinary tract. It is also a good prophylactic for podagra, rheumatism, and hydropsy and is believed to help prevent the formation of kidney stones. This herb has been found to be helpful for both urine incontinence and urine retention. Farmers use it in a cold compress to relieve muscle pain after hard physical labor.

Habitat and collection: Rupturewort is native to southern Europe and Russian Asia. Collect the herb during flowering, between the end of May and early October.

Preparation and dosage: To make an infusion, pour 1 cup (250 ml) of boiling water over 1 tablespoon (15 g) of the herb. Steep for 3 to 5 minutes, cool, and strain. Take 1 tablespoon (15 ml) 4 to 5 times a day after meals.

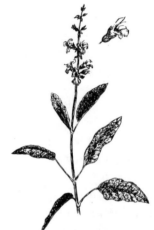

Sage

Botanical name: *Salvia officinalis.*
Family: Labiatae.
Also known as: Red sage, garden sage.

Sage is one of the most popular traditional remedies in Russian herbal medicine and is used to treat a wide variety of common diseases. My family has used sage for generations, both to season food and as a medicinal plant. I remember that when I was a child, my grandmother prepared hot sage tea for me to use as a gargle whenever I had a sore throat.

Sage grows wild but is also cultivated, especially as both a kitchen seasoning and for medicinal use, throughout the Russian Federation. While not native to North America, it is often found in gardens in both the United States and Canada. Cultivated sage has about the same medicinal properties as the wild variety. An ancient proverb states, "How shall a man die who has sage in his garden?"

Part used: Leaves.

Actions: Antihydrotic, antiseptic, antispasmodic, astringent, calmative, expectorant.

Medicinal virtues: Centuries ago, folk healers used sage to heal female sterility. Sage has long been used in folk medicine to cure diseases of the mouth and upper respiratory tract. These uses have been confirmed by official medicine, which recommends the use of sage tea for gargles. A gargle helps relieve symptoms of tonsillitis, sore throat, and laryngitis. Used as a mouthwash, sage tea is used to treat gum infections (gingivitis) and mouth inflammations in general. Official medicine has also found that sage is able to kill certain types of pathogenic organisms and recommends its use to treat skin ulcers and skin inflammation. In a compress, sage is used externally to prevent hair loss and to promote wound healing.

Preparations of sage are taken internally to reduce sweating, especially at night. Sage tea is also used in Russia to decrease the secretion of milk in nursing mothers who wish to wean their babies. Sage tea also increases secretions in the intestinal tract to aid digestion. It is used to treat inflammation of the gallbladder and urinary bladder and to help expel gas from the stomach and intestines.

Habitat and collection: Sage is native to the Mediterranean, but grows throughout Europe and temperate areas of the United States and Canada. Harvest the plant in spring and early summer.

Preparation and dosage: To make a decoction, add 1 teaspoon (15 g) of leaves to 1 cup (250 ml) of boiling water. Lower heat and simmer gently for 30 minutes, then cool for 30 minutes at room temperature. Filter. Take 2 to 3 tablespoons (30 to 45 ml) 3 to 4 times a day for 7 to 10 days.

To prepare an infusion, add 1 teaspoon (5 g) of leaves to 1½ cups (400 ml) of boiling water. Turn off the heat and allow to stand for 20 to 30 minutes. Filter. Take ¼ cup (60 ml) 3 to 4 times a day with meals. The course of treatment is 1 to 12 days.

Caution: **Sage tea should be avoided during pregnancy. If used in excess (or over long periods of time), sage can cause symptoms of poisoning. Do not exceed 1 cup of the infusion per day and limit the course of treatment to 14 days per month.**

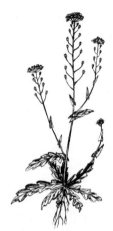

SHEPHERD'S PURSE

Botanical name: *Capsella bursa-pastoris.*
Family: Cruciferae.
Also known as: St. James's weed, pickpocket.

The name *shepherd's purse* came about for two reasons: the shape of the seeds (flat, triangular, and with a heart-shaped notch on the top) is reminiscent of the purses shepherds used to carry with them as they tended their flocks, and traveling shepherds often carried this useful herb in their purses. As a medicinal remedy, shepherd's purse has enjoyed a wide variety of applications since early Greek and Roman times. Traces of this herb have also been found in archaeological digs in territories where early Slavic tribes once thrived.

During the Middle Ages, shepherd's purse was used by peasants living throughout Russia and much of Europe primarily to stop bleeding but it was later largely forgotten except among folk healers. In imperial Russia, official medicine rediscovered the benefits of this herb during the First World War, when there was a strong interest in finding simple remedies that could stop the bleeding of wounds. Additional research later revealed a number of other useful medicinal properties of this ancient herb, which now enjoys a prominent place in Russian official medicine.

Parts used: Aerial parts.

Actions: Antisclerotic, diuretic, hemostatic, stimulant, vasoconstrictor.

Medicinal virtues: As a powerful hemostatic, an infusion of shepherd's purse is recommended to treat symptoms of internal bleeding, including that of the stomach (gastrorrhagia), the kidneys (nephrorragia), larynx (laryngorragia), and the nose (rhinorrhagia).

Shepherd's purse infusions or extracts increase the tone of the uterus and the smooth muscles of the intestine. For this reason, Russian herbalists recommend this herb to improve uterine tone and to counteract excessive or difficult menstruation.

As a styptic, a decoction or fresh juice is often prescribed to treat acute or chronic diseases of the intestine, including stomach and duodenal ulcers. Shepherd's purse is also effective for treating catarrhal diseases, rheumatism, sclerosis, piles, and ague.

In folk medicine, an infusion of this herb (as well as the juice) is used to treat diseases of the kidney, gallbladder, urinary bladder, and liver. It is also used to treat gastritis, hypertension, gestational toxosis, and nausea. This herb has a tendency to narrow the peripheral blood vessels and is used to increase blood pressure and normalize heartbeat.

Because it contains numerous trace minerals, including copper, zinc, manganese, and chromium, shepherd's purse is an effective remedy for disbolism, including diabetes.

In dermatology, shepherd's purse infusions or juice are used externally to treat vasculitis, eczema, hemorrhoids, wounds, and cuts.

Habitat and collection: It is believed that this herb is of European or west Asiatic origin, although it grows throughout the nontropical world. Collect the herb from March through October.

Preparation and dosage: To make an infusion, add 1 cup (250 ml) of hot water to 1 tablespoon (15 g) of the dried herb in a container. Allow to steep for 15 minutes and strain. Take 1 tablespoon (15 ml) 3 to 4 times a day, 20 minutes before meals.

To make a cold extract, soak 1 tablespoon (15 g) of fresh herb in ³/₄ cup (200 ml) of cold water. Allow to stand for 8 to 10 hours. Take 2 tablespoons (30 ml) 3 times a day.

Prepare a juice according to the directions given in "Making Herbal Preparations," but dilute with an equal part of water and do not heat. Take 1 teaspoon (5 ml) 3 to 4 times a day.

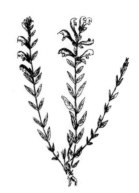

SKULLCAP

Botanical name: *Scutellaria baicalensis.*
Family: Labiatae.
Also known as: Helmet flower,
　blue pimpernel.

The use of skullcap traces its origins to the early inhabitants who lived in eastern Siberia, especially near the shores of Lake Baikal, Russia's deepest and most beautiful lake. It is believed that knowledge of this herb originally came from China, where herbalists called it *huantesin.* Since skullcap grows in many parts of the world (there are three hundred known varieties of this herb), it has become a major part of most folk-healing traditions.

Russian official medicine took notice of skullcap in the 1950s when early research was undertaken by scientists at the western Siberian branch of the Academy of Sciences of the Soviet Union. Additional research was done at the University of Tomsk School of Medicine, making skullcap one of Russia's most thoroughly investigated herbs by the late 1980s.

Parts used: Aerial parts, roots.

Actions: Anthelmintic, antihypertensive, antiphlogistic, antipyretic, antispasmodic, calmative, cholagogue, diuretic, hemostatic, purgative, sedative, tonic.

Medicinal virtues: In official herbal medicine, a skullcap infusion is prescribed to treat the initial stages of hypertension, and regular use is believed to reduce blood pressure and slow down the heart rhythm. As a sedative, skullcap is a good remedy to treat neurosis and other diseases of the nervous system. It has also been used to relieve headache, tinnitus, chest pain, and insomnia. It is recommended for treating disorders of the liver and gastrointestinal tract, as well as epilepsy, rheumatism, bronchitis, and whooping cough. Herbalists also use skullcap infusions to increase the appetite and to treat symptoms of cold and flu.

Habitat and collection: Skullcap is native to wet places in western Russia, the northern United States, and southern Canada. The flowering plant can be collected from August to September.

Preparation and dosage: To prepare an infusion, add 1 cup (250 ml) of hot water to 1 teaspoon (5 g) of dried herb. Steep for 30 minutes. Filter. Take 1 cup 3 to 4 times daily.

To make a tincture, put 1 ounce (40 g) of fresh, chopped roots or $^1/_2$ ounce (20 g) of dried, crushed roots in 1 cup (250 ml) of 70-proof alcohol. Keep for 15 days in a tightly closed container in a dark place. Shake daily. Filter. Take $^3/_4$ teaspoon (3 ml) 3 times a day.

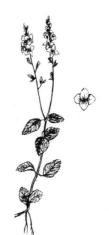

SPEEDWELL
Botanical name: *Veronica officinalis*
Family: Scrophulariaceae.
Also known as: Gypsy weed, veronica.

The name for speedwell in the Russian language means "Anita's eyes." In Russian folklore, Anita fell in love with a young man who would declare his love to every pretty girl in town only to abandon her later for someone new. Anita had very beautiful eyes and told the man that if he ever found someone new, her eyes would follow him everywhere. The man didn't pay attention to her words and, as usual, told her that she was his only true love. He then went to visit another young woman but felt that Anita's eyes were indeed following him everywhere he walked. He decided to come back to Anita and never strayed again.

Speedwell possesses a rich variety of healing properties and is used either alone or with other herbs to treat a wide range of health conditions. However, its exact chemical composition has not yet been completely researched.

Healing preparations from speedwell have been used in Russia for centuries. In some areas of Russia, speedwell was used primarily to treat snakebite and was therefore known as "snake's herb." In other parts, it was used to treat lung and bronchial problems and was therefore called "the chest herb."

Parts used: Flowers, leaves.

Actions: Appetizer, calmative, digestive, diuretic, hemostatic, stomachic, tonic.

Medicinal virtues: Speedwell preparations are used to treat diseases of the stomach and the intestinal tract, such as diarrhea. An infusion of this herb stimulates the appetite and aids digestion. An effective expectorant, speedwell is also used to treat diseases of the respiratory tract like cough, bronchial asthma, and hoarseness. Taken internally, the infusion is used for podagra (gout, especially of the joints of the foot), gallstones, and kidney stones. It is also taken hot to soothe intestinal colic, relieve headache, calm nervousness, and treat insomnia.

Many folk healers use speedwell either alone or in combination with other herbs, such as pansy, black elder, or ground ivy, to treat eczema, skin rashes, and certain fungal infections. Externally, speedwell infusions are used to stop bleeding and to treat genital itching among older women, especially if they have diabetes. In Russia, ointments made with speedwell are used to treat sunburn and chronic skin problems. Fresh leaves that have been soaked in water can also be applied to the skin to treat burns and wounds. The juice can also be used to wash wounds and to treat sunburn or fungal infections.

Habitat and collection: Speedwell is originally from the Caucasus and grows in fields, woods, and meadows throughout Russia and Europe. The flowers are collected from June through August.

Preparation and dosage: To make an infusion, add 1 cup (250 ml) of boiling water to 1 tablespoon (15 g) of herb. Allow to stand for 10 minutes at room temperature. Filter. Take ¼ to ⅓ cup (60 to 80 ml) 4 times daily after meals.

Prepare a juice using the directions given in "Making Herbal Preparations." For internal use, add 2 to 3 teaspoons (5 to 15 ml) of the juice to water or milk and drink in the morning before eating. (Folk healers recommend that you add 2 to 3 teaspoons (5 to 15 ml) of goat milk to the juice instead.) Use the juice externally for washing wounds and for treating sunburn or fungal infections.

———

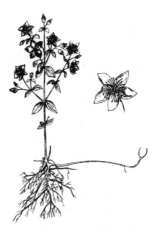

St. Johnswort

Botanical name: *Hypericum perforatum.*
Family: Hypericaceae.
Also known as: Amber, goatweed.

According to an old Russian proverb, "It is as impossible to make bread without flour as it is to heal people without St. Johnswort." This herb was so popular in early Russia that Czar Michael I issued a special order that no less than one hundred pounds of this herb be collected each year to be delivered to the court. Throughout the rest of northern Europe, St. Johnswort has an ancient reputation for protecting humans from evil spirits, because a whiff of it made the spirits fly away. In Russia St. Johnswort was believed to protect humans from dangerous forest animals, possibly because hunters observed that animals who ate this herb eventually became ill. Earlier in this century, Russian scientists noted that St. Johnswort contains a special pigment that can make some animals, including humans, very sensitive to sunshine. When an animal is affected in this way, it often throws itself on the ground and tends to bite the sensitive places. Although St. Johnswort is still regarded as an important medicinal herb today, it can produce supersensitivity to sunlight in some people.

Parts used: Aerial parts.

Actions: Anodyne, antiseptic, antispasmodic, astringent, expectorant, vulnerary.

Medicinal virtues: Preparations of St. Johnswort promote the flow of urine, and the filtration of urine by the kidneys. They also promote the expulsion of bile from the gallbladder and are used to relieve a variety of pulmonary complaints.

A decoction of this herb is used to treat gout and rheumatism, as well as diseases of the stomach, kidneys, and intestinal tract.

An infusion of St. Johnswort is beneficial (as an anodyne) for both headaches and pains in the eyes that are related to overexcitement and nervousness. It is also prescribed in Russia for people suffering from insomnia, chest congestion, tuberculosis, and hemorrhoids.

The oil extract is an old folk remedy applied externally to treat burns, sores, and wounds, while a tincture is used as a gargle to treat sores in the gums and mouth.

Habitat and collection: St. Johnswort is found in meadows and woods throughout northern Europe, Asia, and North America. The flowers bloom from June to August and all aerial parts can be harvested during these months.

Preparation and dosage: To make a decoction, place 1 tablespoon (5 g) of herb into 1 cup (250 ml) of water. Simmer over low heat for 30 minutes. Cool for 10 minutes, filter, and squeeze. Take ⅓ cup (80 ml) 3 times a day a half hour before mealtimes. Once prepared, the decoction is good for no more than 3 days. A course of treatment can last for 2 to 3 weeks.

To make an infusion, add 1 teaspoon (5 g) of herb to 1 cup (250 ml) of hot water. Cover and steep for 5 minutes. Take ½ cup (125 ml) 30 minutes before breakfast and another ½ cup (125 ml) 30 minutes before going to bed. A recommended course of treatment ranges from 2 to 3 weeks.

To make an oil extract, mix 2 tablespoons (30 g) of finely chopped fresh flowers and 1 teaspoon (5 g) of chopped fresh leaves with 1 cup (250 ml) of vegetable oil. Cover and let stand for 2 to 3 weeks, stirring it daily. Filter through 2 to 3 layers of cotton gauze. Use the extract on sore or infected skin.

To make a tincture, mix 3 ounces (100 g) of dried herb with 1½ cups (400 ml) of 80-proof vodka. Let stand for 3 days in a tightly closed glass jar. Use 30 to 40 drops in ½ cup (125 ml) of warm water as a gargle. If taken internally, place 20 drops in 1 cup of water, and take once a day before eating. A course of treatment can continue for 1 to 2 weeks.

———

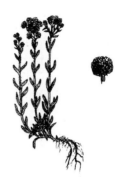

STRAWFLOWER

Botanical name: *Helichrysum arenarium.*
Family: Compositae.
Also known as: Eternal flower.

In old Russia this herb was known as "the immortalizer." According to old fairy tales, this herb can make you immortal if you are lucky enough to find a blue blossom on this plant in sandy or rocky soil, near sand dunes, or in a field. Fairy tales aside, this plant has a yellow flower and is not guaranteed to make one immortal. Yet the English nickname for this plant, "eternal flower," gives some indication of its wonderful medicinal properties. It is one of the most widely used herbs in Russia today.

Parts used: Flowers.

Actions: Anthelmintic, antilithic, disinfectant, hemostatic.

Medicinal virtues: Herbal preparations made with strawflower improve bile secretion, reduce the secretion of acid by the liver, improve gallbladder function, help activate the adrenal glands, and increase the production and elimination of urine. It may also be used to eliminate certain types of ascaris, an intestinal worm.

Russian doctors prescribe an infusion of strawflower to break up small gallstones and help eliminate them from the gallbladder. It is also recommended for treatment of cholecystitis (inflammation of the gallbladder), hepatitis, gastritis, and liver problems. The official commercial herbal preparation known as Flamin (derived from the flavenoids of the *Helichrysum arenarium*) is prescribed for chronic cholecystitis and hepaticholecystitis.

An infusion of this herb is also used to help relieve chronic inflammation of the kidneys resulting in difficulty passing urine. It is used to disinfect the kidneys and increase urine excretion. It also helps relieve low-acid gastritis and liver problems accompanied by colic or spasm.

Habitat and collection: This flower blooms between June and October. Harvest only flowers that have recently opened.

Preparation and dosage: To make an infusion for chronic kidney inflammation, add 1 tablespoon (15 g) of dried flowers to 1 cup (250 ml) of boiling water. Cover, steep for 10 to 15 minutes, and then strain. Take ¹/₂ cup (125 ml) per day 15 minutes before a meal. Continue dosage for 2 to 3 weeks.

To make an extract of *Helicrysum arenarium,* add 3 tablespoons (45 g) of dried flowers in a pot containing 1 cup (250 ml) of water. Cover the pot loosely and simmer the mixture for 3 minutes. Let cool for 10 minutes at room temperature and strain. Take ¹/₂ cup (125 ml) 2 to 3 times a day 15 minutes before eating.

———

THYME

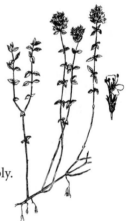

Botanical name: *Thymus serpellum.*
Family: Labiatae.
Also known as: Garden thyme *(Thymus vulgaris),*
 which is very similar in appearance,
 actions, and medical virtues to
 Thymus serpellum but is somewhat
 stronger. Both herbs can be used interchangeably.

Thyme is one of the best-known traditional Russian herbal plants and was known for centuries as "our lady's herb." In addition to its use as a folk remedy, the leaves were added to sacrificial holy fires by Slavic tribes before the advent of Christianity. They considered the aromatic smoke a sign that the sacrifice was accepted by the gods. After early Russians were converted to Christianity some ten centuries ago, the sacred use of this herb in religious ceremonies continued but was primarily expressed by using thyme to decorate icons of the Virgin Mary on the Holy Day of Our Lady, celebrated in late August according to the Russian Orthodox Church.

Parts used: Aerial parts.

Actions: Analgesic, antimicrobial, antispasmodic, astringent, carminative, expectorant, tonic.

Medicinal virtues: An extract of thyme is a part of Pertusin, an officially produced medicine in the former Soviet Union for bronchitis and whooping cough. Thyme oil is used in making Thymol, used to disinfect the mucous membrane of the mouth and throat and to soothe the processes of fermentation in the intestines. Thymol is also effective in alleviating symptoms of diarrhea.

 An extract of thyme makes up a part of the so-called Gartman's mixture, used in dental practice to relieve tooth pain. It is also good when added to a bath for sore joints, and a 10 percent solution is used to eliminate fungal diseases of the skin. When taken internally, the solution is reputed to alleviate symptoms of antinomycosis, a fungal disease in farm animals that is sometimes transmitted to humans.

Official Russian medicine approves of thyme for a wide range of health problems that have long been treated by traditional folk healers. Russian physicians prescribe thyme for spasm in the stomach, neuralgia, insomnia, and for respiratory and digestive infections. It is also used as a gargle for laryngitis and tonsillitis. As an expectorant, thyme is used to help alleviate coughs, bronchitis, and asthma. It is often prescribed for bed-wetting and childhood diarrhea. Doctors also recommend aromatic baths of thyme for relaxation and for stimulating digestion. A cool thyme extract is perfect to wash sore eyes, and herbalists prepare a cold compress containing thyme to relieve eye soreness and discomfort. They wash the scalp with thyme extract to ease headaches and use an infusion of thyme as a shampoo to relieve dandruff.

An infusion of thyme is taken externally for itchiness, rashes, skin infections, and wounds. Old folk healers also placed dried thyme leaves and flowers in pillows to facilitate sleep and to prevent colds. Extract of thyme has been used to help people break the alcohol habit, but Russians have developed a more effective remedy using thyme in conjunction with other herbs, which can be found in the section of complex herbal recipes.

Habitat and collection: Thyme is naturally found throughout Europe and North America. It is also extensively cultivated in gardens throughout the world. Harvest from late May through September.

Preparation and dosage: For internal use, prepare an infusion by adding 2 tablespoons (30 g) of dry herb to 2 cups (500 ml) of boiling water. Steep for 1 hour, filter, and cool to room temperature. Take ¹/₂ cup (125 ml) 3 times a day before eating. A course of treatment should not be longer than 4 weeks.

To make a cool extract for sore eyes, boil 4 tablespoons (60 g) of dry herb or 2 tablespoons (30 g) of fresh thyme in 1 quart (1 liter) of water. Cool to room temperature. Soak a cloth or towel in the infusion, wring out, and place over the eyes.

As a bath additive, add 3 ounces (100 g) of dry herb into 2 quarts (2 liters) of boiling water. Steep for 30 minutes in a warm place and filter. This mixture may also be used as a gargle.

Caution: **Do not exceed recommended dosage. Excessive internal use of thyme can overstimulate the thyroid gland and lead to symptoms of poisoning.**

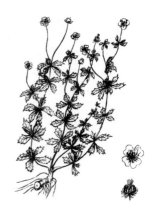

TORMENTIL
Botanical name: *Tormentilla erecta* or
  Potentilla tormentilla.
Family: Rosaceae.
Also known as: Shepherd's knot.

Tormentil has been a very popular herbal remedy in Russia for centuries. During the Middle Ages, the herb was given the Latin name *Potentilla tormentilla; tormentilla* comes from *tormina,* the Latin word for dysentery, and *pontentilla* comes from *potentia,* meaning "power." It later became a part of Russian official medicine and became known under its more accepted Latin name, *Tormentilla erecta.*

Parts used: Rootstocks.

Actions: Antiphlogistic, antiseptic, astringent, hemostatic, styptic.

Medicinal virtues: Tormentil is widely used in both folk and official medicine in Russia. A tormentil infusion is often recommended for treating diseases of the gastrointestinal tract, including enteritis (intestinal catarrh), colitis, dyspepsia, and dysentery. It is especially beneficial for people with intestinal problems that include diarrhea or constipation. It is also useful for relieving symptoms of stomach and duodenal ulcers. Folk healers use tormentil infusions for tuberculosis, emphysema, and anemia. In addition, it is recommended for podagra, rheumatism, and jaundice. A decoction made from tormentil promotes the onset of menstruation.

A tormentil infusion makes a good mouthwash and gargle for treating sore throat, laryngitis, and inflammation of the mucous membranes in the mouth, including bleeding gums and mouth sores. In dermatology, it is taken internally to relieve symptoms of vasculitis and is used externally as a compress for wounds, bruises, eczema, burns, and neurodermatitis. It is also good for healing chapped and splitting skin.

Habitat and collection: Tormentil is found primarily in pastures, meadows, and marshes. Dig up the root in early autumn.

Preparation and dosage: To make an infusion, add 1 cup (250 ml) of boiling water to 1 tablespoon (15 g) of chopped rootstocks. Steep for 30 minutes, strain, and store at room temperature. Take ¼ cup (60 ml) 4 to 5 times a day 30 minutes before meals.

To prepare a decoction, add 2 tablespoons (30 g) of roots to 1 cup (250 ml) of boiling water. Simmer on low heat for 15 minutes. Strain. Take 1 tablespoon (15 ml) 4 to 5 times a day 30 minutes before meals.

To make a mouthwash, dilute the decoction with water (1 part decoction to 4 parts water). Take every 2 hours.

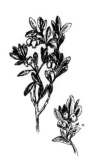

Uva Ursi
Botanical name: *Arctostaphylos uva-ursi.*
Family: Ericaceae.
Also known as: Bearberry, kinnikinnick.

Uva ursi is called "bear's ear" or "bear's berry" in Russia. For those who understand the nuances of the Russian language, these names (along with "rabbit's grass" or "wolf's berry") indicate that the plant is not fit for human consumption because it is either foul tasting or poisonous and yet often visually attractive.

Such is the case with uva ursi berries, which bear a close resemblance to good Alpine cranberries. However, let only the bears eat them! Fortunately, humans have discovered ways to use the leaves of this plant to effectively treat a wide variety of health problems.

Parts used: Leaves.

Actions: Anodyne, antiphlogistic, antiseptic, astringent, cardiac, demulcent, depurative, diuretic, tonic.

Medicinal virtues: Russian herbalists recommend an uva ursi decoction to treat inflammation of the bladder, kidney, and urinary tract. It has also been found to relieve the pain of bladder stones and gravel due to urolithiasis. Official Russian herbal doctors prescribe uva ursi for gynecological infections and diseases of the gastrointestinal tract, including chronic constipation and indigestion. It is also an effective treatment for cardiac insufficiency and liver problems. A decoction made from uva ursi is prescribed for suppurative wounds, sores, and diathesis. In folk medicine, a decoction is used to treat bronchitis, asthma, and colds.

Herbalists prescribe infusions to treat tuberculosis and diabetes and regard it as an effective remedy for treating nervousness and alcoholism. As an anodyne, uva ursi helps relieve rheumatic pains. It is also used to treat podagra.

Habitat and collection: This shrub is found throughout central Russia, southern Canada, and in the northern parts of the United States. The leaves of this evergreen are best collected in spring and early summer.

Preparation and dosage: To make an infusion, add 1 cup (250 ml) of boiling water to 1 teaspoon (5 g) of dried leaves. Cover and steep for 10 to 15 minutes and strain. Drink 1 cup (250 ml) 3 times daily.

To prepare a decoction, add 1 tablespoon (5 g) of dried leaves to 1 cup (250 ml) of water. Heat to a boil then simmer gently for 10 minutes. Strain. Take ¼ cup (60 ml) up to 3 times a day for no more than 20 days.

To prepare a tincture, soak 2 teaspoons (3 g) of dried leaves in ½ cup (125 ml) of 40-proof spirits in a warm place for 15 days. Strain. Take 10 to 15 drops 3 times a day after meals for no more than 4 weeks.

Caution: **Do not exceed recommended dosage. Excessive doses of bearberry can lead to stomach distress, while prolonged use can result in chronic poisoning. It should be avoided by pregnant women. Do not consume the berries.**

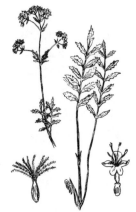

Valerian
Botanical name: *Valeriana officinalis.*
Family: Valerianaceae.
Also known as: Fragrant valerian.

Fragrant valerian has been a well-known and widely used herb in Russia for nearly two thousand years. According to an old Russian legend, the folk healer (and later, a saint) Panteleimon went into the forest one day to pick herbs. Because nightfall was quickly approaching, Panteleimon decided to leave the forest. He suddenly saw hundreds of light pink shimmering lights that appeared on the ground like moving currents of color. These streams were made of small blue clouds that looked like flowers. Panteleimon then began digging up the roots. When he had acquired a bagful of roots, his soul was filled with joy. He went from village to village and gave the roots to sick people telling them to "be healthy." The legend goes on to say that this herb can be used to treat a wide range of diseases.

Parts used: Rootstocks.

Actions: Antispasmodic, calmative, carminative, hypnotic, nervine, sedative, stomachic.

Medicinal virtues: In Russian folk and official medicine, valerian is used as a calmative and anodyne to treat nervousness and anxiety, migraine headaches, insomnia, hysteria, epileptic fits, neuralgia, skeletal muscle spasms, and nervous spasm of the stomach and intestines. Both the infusion and cold extract help ease menstrual cramps. Recent Russian research has found that infusions made with fragrant valerian can treat diseases of the thyroid gland. Valerian is often used to treat insomnia, either alone or combined with chamomile, passionflower, and hops.

In general, preparations made from valerian are believed to cause no adverse side effects. However, if taken in excessive doses, it may produce intestinal problems and cause drowsiness and lack of alertness. When discontinued, symptoms quickly disappear. Generally speaking, herbalists recommend that valerian preparations not be taken more than once or twice per day for a period of 3 weeks. We recommend limiting the course of treatment to 2 months per year.

Habitat and collection: Native to Europe and Asia, valerian favors shady, wooded, and slightly damp places such as marshes. The best time to harvest the root is in late August or September.

Preparation and dosage: To make an infusion, add 1 tablespoon (15 g) of dry rootstocks to 1 cup (250 ml) of boiling water. Cover, let steep for 15 minutes, and strain. Take 1 cup (250 ml) 3 times a day after meals.

To prepare a cold extract for treating menstrual cramps, add 1 cup (250 ml) of boiling water to 1 teaspoon (5 g) of dried, powdered roots. Allow to stand for 2 hours. Take $^1/_2$ cup (125 ml) in the morning and another $^1/_2$ cup (125 ml) before bedtime.

To make a tincture, add 2 tablespoons (30 g) of dried, powdered roots to $^1/_2$ cup (125 ml) of 90-proof alcohol mixed with $^1/_2$ cup (125 ml) of water. Bring to a boil. Cover and allow to stand for 2 weeks at room temperature. Stir twice daily. Pour the liquid into another bottle through a filter. Squeeze the excess liquid from the roots into the new bottle and discard the roots. Filter mixture once more. Add 15 drops of this tincture to a cup of water and drink 3 times a day.

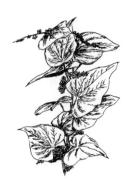

WILD YAM
Botanical name: *Dioscorea villosa.*
Family: Dioscoreaceae.

There are up to five hundred herbs belonging to the Dioscoreaceae family, including *Dioscorea caucasia, Dioscorea nipponica,* and *Dioscorea deltoides.* Many of these herbs have attracted the attention of Russian scientists because they contain a steroid known as *saponin,* a valuable and effective substitute for steroid hormones in treating a number of diseases. One of the best sources for saponin is the wild yam, which has been cultivated on small farms in Russia for many years.

Before saponin was discovered in wild yam, pharmaceutical companies had to extract the hormone from the glands of cattle. The discovery of the steroid substitute in wild yam provided a more humane and sanitary alternative to this practice.

European and American herbalists have been using wild yam for many years, although vitamin and pharmaceutical companies have only recently been exploring its medicinal properties. By contrast, in Russia a commercial preparation known as Polysporin, made from saponin from *Discorea nipponica,* used to treat arteriosclerosis, was approved by Russian official medicine decades ago.

Parts used: Roots.

Actions: Anticoagulant, antisclerotic, antispasmodic, cholagogue, depurative, diaphoretic, diuretic, vasodilator.

Medicinal virtues: Russian scientists prepare saponin extracts from the roots of different varieties of wild yam and use these preparations for reducing levels of serum cholesterol and blood pressure. Saponin appears to help certain proteins (known as *albumens*) to hold cholesterol in colloidal suspension, which prevents it from sticking to arterial walls. It is also used for treating intestinal colic, diverticulitis, and rheumatoid arthritis. People like wild yam because it is both natural and effective and causes no adverse side effects. In addition, patients have reported improved memory, better sleep, and an overall feeling of increased well-being. Some folk herbalists recommend infusions of wild yam for treating nervous conditions, neuralgia, and pain in the urinary tract. For people suffering from one or more of the conditions described in this paragraph, wild yam may be the most effective natural remedy one can use.

For some individuals, wild yam preparations can cause slight stomach irritation, so Russian herbalists often recommend that they be taken after meals. Except for this minor side effect, no adverse reactions have been found.

Habitat and collection: This herb is widely cultivated. Collect the roots in autumn.

Preparation and dosage: To prepare a decoction, put 1 tablespoon (15 g) of chopped or crushed dried roots in an enameled metal or heatproof glass pot. Add 1 cup (250 ml) of boiling water. Cover the pot. The water and roots should not fill more than ¹/₃ of the container's volume. Simmer on low heat for 30 minutes, and cool at room temperature for another 45 minutes. Strain and add more boiling water until the mixture reaches its original 1 cup (250 ml).

Take 1 tablespoon (15 ml) 3 times a day after meals. The entire course of treatment should consist of 3 to 4 cycles. Each cycle should last from 20 to 30 days, with a break of 7 to 10 days between cycles.

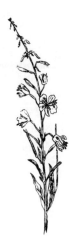

WILLOW HERB
Botanical name: *Chamaenerion* or
　Epilobium angustifolium.
Family: Onagracae.
Also known as: Rosebay willow herb,
　fireweed.

This tall, beautiful perennial, known as "Ivan's tea" centuries ago, was once Russia's most popular nonalcoholic beverage, often enjoyed as a refreshing hot drink after meals. Nearly every peasant family grew Ivan's tea in their garden. But after Chinese black tea was introduced to the continent, they abandoned their efforts. However, residents in the town of Kapor continued to grow it, which is one reason why this plant is also known today as "Kaporic tea."

As a caffeine-free beverage, willow herb is relaxing and calmative. Although modern Russians prefer black tea for everyday use, they value Ivan's tea for its medicinal properties.

Parts used: Flowers, leaves.

Actions: Antiphlogistic, antispasmodic, astringent, calmative, demulcent, styptic.

Medicinal virtues: As a calmative, an infusion made from the leaves of this herb is used to relieve headaches and promote sleep. A decoction made from willow herb is used as a styptic and antiphlogistic for stomach and intestinal problems such as ulcers, colitis, and gastritis. It is also used to relieve symptoms of scrofula. In folk medicine, a powder made from willow herb is used to heal wounds, and a poultice of willow is an effective remedy to treat inflammation of the ears, throat, and nose. Willow herb can also be used to relieve asthma episodes and to treat whooping cough and hiccoughs.

Habitat and collection: This healing herb grows in open woodlands, waste places, slag heaps, and barren areas throughout Europe, western Asia, and North America. Because it tends to crowd out other plants, willow herb is often unpopular with herb gardeners. Collect the herb in midsummer when in bloom.

Preparation and dosage: To make a decoction, soak 1 tablespoon (15 g) of leaves in 1 cup (250 ml) of cold water. Heat to boiling then simmer for 15 minutes. Allow to stand for 2 hours and strain. Take 1 tablespoon (15 ml) 4 times a day before meals.

To make an infusion, add 1 teaspoon (10 g) of dried leaves or flowers to 1 cup (250 ml) of boiling water. Cover and steep for 15 minutes before straining. Take 1 cup (250 ml) twice a day (after lunch and at bedtime) to normalize minor stomach disorders.

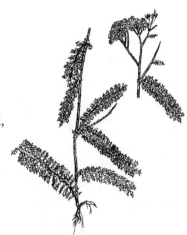

YARROW

Botanical name: *Achillea millefolium.*
Family: Compositae.
Also known as: Milfoil, thousand weed,
  nosebleed.

Yarrow is one of our most ancient medicinal plants and is mentioned in Greek mythology. The herb received its name, which eventually became the botanical name *Achillea,* from the hero Achilles. He used the herb to heal the wounds he received in his famous battle with Telefus. Because it has often been used to stop bleeding, early Europeans called it "soldier's wound wort" and "knight's milfoil."

Russians call yarrow the "herb of a thousand leaves." Old herbals document its medicinal use in Russia as far back as the fourteenth century, although it was probably used before that time. During the eighteenth and nineteenth centuries, Russian doctors were very familiar with the medicinal properties of yarrow and used it to treat hemorrhage and relieve symptoms of dysentery.

In some Eastern European countries like Hungary and Poland, yarrow is used in the manufacture of modern pharmaceuticals. Russians tend to adhere to a more natural approach and market it primarily in the form of extracts and infusions.

Parts used: Aerial parts.

Actions: Antiphlogistic, antiseptic, antispasmodic, appetizer, astringent, carminative, cholagogue, coagulant, diaphoretic, hemostatic, tonic.

Medicinal virtues: Yarrow contains a chemical substance known as *achellein,* which increases the ability of the blood to clot 60 percent more efficiently than the compound calcium chloride, often used in allopathic medicine. Yarrow is often used by Russian folk herbalists to stop internal bleeding, especially in the lungs and stomach. It is also used to stop nasal and hemorrhoidal bleeding. Herbalists consider yarrow the herb of choice to stop uterine bleeding during menstruation, because in addition to the herb's property as a coagulant, it has also been found to strengthen the muscles of the uterus. This herb is also recommended for nursing mothers who wish to increase lactation.

Russian herbalists claim that yarrow acts as a relaxant for the muscles of the intestines and urinary tract and reduces meteorism. They often recommend yarrow juice, decoctions, or extracts to treat gastritis, stomach ulcers, and duodenal ulcers, as well as to stimulate the appetite and reduce flatulence. Yarrow is also believed to reduce blood pressure, stimulate the flow of liver bile (which is used to digest fats), and guard against the formation of kidney stones and gallstones.

Since ancient times, yarrow has been employed to treat a variety of skin problems. Preparations made with fresh yarrow juice and olive oil are used in a compress by folk healers to treat furunculosis, skin tuberculosis, sore hands, sore nipples, and excessive hair loss. Herbalists also combine external yarrow preparations with infusions taken internally. Yarrow infusions are also used externally to wash wounds, burns, and skin ulcers. Fresh yarrow juice, applied directly to the scalp, is recommended for excessive hair loss.

Habitat and collection: Yarrow grows wild in sunny meadows, pastures, and along roadsides throughout Europe and much of North America. Gather the herb after flowering, between June and October.

Preparation and dosage: To make a compress, mix 1 part of fresh yarrow juice with 10 parts of olive oil. Use as a cold compress to treat skin problems. Change once daily.

To prepare a tincture, take 3 tablespoons (45 g) of dried powdered herb combined with 10 ounces (30 ml) of 90-proof alcohol. Allow to stand for three days. Add 50 percent distilled water, and allow to stand for 2 weeks, shaking the mixture once or twice a week. Strain and store in a dark-colored bottle with a secure cap. Take 40 to 50 drops 3 times a day before meals to treat uterine bleeding caused by inflammation and excessive menstrual flow.

To make a decoction, add 2 tablespoons (30 g) of dried herb to 1 cup (250 ml) of hot water. Bring to a boil and simmer gently for 15 minutes. Allow to cool for 45 minutes at room temperature. Strain. Take $1/2$ cup (125 ml) 2 to 3 times a day 30 minutes before meals.

To prepare a juice for external application, use fresh aerial parts and follow the directions given in "Making Herbal Preparations."

Caution: Long-term use of yarrow (i.e., 2 months or more) can make the skin sensitive to sunlight.

COMPLEX
HERBAL FORMULAS

In addition to using single herbs for healing, Russian healers have discovered that certain herbal combinations can enhance the healing process. Through generations of experimentation and use, they developed hundreds of complex herbal formulas that offer several advantages over single herbal preparations.

Herbal formulas can be very powerful. Because many of the herbs used have synergetic effects, which makes the combination more powerful than its component parts, the formulas also tend to react faster and their effects are more complete than if the herbs are used alone.

In addition, different herbs used in proper combinations and amounts often support a number of body organs and functions at the same time. Since certain groups of organs in the body work very closely together—such as the liver and the kidneys—the overall effects of the herbal formula are enhanced. A complex recipe may act on a variety of organs and tissues that may be affected by a specific health problem. For example, a formula may help lower blood pressure and promote restful sleep. In addition, one group of symptoms is often accompanied by related symptoms from another health problem. Many of the complex recipes are able to deal with both diseases at the same time.

Although most of the herbs presented in this book can be used alone, complex herbal recipes offer more specific healing properties than single plants. The recipes represent two major goals of the Russian school of herbalism: to use as few ingredients in a recipe as possible, while producing maximum therapeutic effect (by contrast, formulas made according to the Arabic tradition of herbalism can involve a dozen different herbs or more); and to not only pinpoint the main disease symptoms, but to address associated symptoms as well.

The herbal formulas presented in this section are based on many years of clinical use by both official and folk herbalists in Russia. Many of these formulas have gone through the same rigorous laboratory and clinical trials undertaken for a commercially prepared allopathic drug.

To prepare these herbal remedies at home, choose good quality herbs and follow the general directions given in the chapter "Making Herbal Preparations." If a recipe does not call for a specific part of an herb, use the aerial parts.

Home diagnosis, however, is not advised. All diseases should be diagnosed by a qualified health-care professional. Many diseases may be the result of other conditions or the symptoms of a particular disease may be similar to those of another.

The Digestive Organs

❦

In digestion the body breaks down proteins, starches, and fats both mechanically and chemically in the gastrointestinal tract, where they are converted into smaller molecules that the body can absorb. Many different parts of the body are involved in digestion, including the mouth, stomach, colon, small intestine, and the pancreas and other glands. Saliva, gastric juice, and pancreatic juice promote digestion, while bile emulsifies fats.

Digestive disorders are very common, and in addition to diet, exercise, stress reduction, and medications, a wide variety of herbal treatments have been developed to treat many common digestive problems. On the following pages, we will examine some diseases of the digestive organs and how complex herbal formulas may help in their treatment.

Stomatitis

Stomatitis is a clinical term describing inflammation of the mouth. It often manifests as increased production of saliva, bad breath, heat, pain, and fever. It is often due to viruses and bacteria, but can also be caused by irritants like hot or spicy food, tobacco smoke, chemicals in toothpastes and other products, nutritional deficiencies, and systemic infections including measles and syphilis.

Since the causes and symptoms of stomatitis vary, diagnosis determines which specific herbal formula is used. The following complex remedies are used only to complement traditional medical therapy and in that capacity have been found to be very effective.

STOMATITIS RECIPE 1

> 2 parts oak bark   1 part St. Johnswort
> 1 part sage leaves

Place 1¹/₂ teaspoons (7 g) of herbal mixture in a water banya and add 1 cup (250 ml) of hot water. Simmer for 15 minutes over low heat. Turn off heat and steep for 45 minutes. Strain. Use as a gargle for up to 5 minutes every hour during the day.

STOMATITIS RECIPE 2

> 2 parts chamomile flowers   2 parts peppermint leaves
> 3 parts sage leaves   1 part fennel seeds

Prepare and take as above.

STOMATITIS RECIPE 3

> 4 parts oak bark   2 parts althaea roots
> 4 parts marjoram   3 parts elecampane roots

Prepare and take as above.

STOMATITIS RECIPE 4

> 1 part chamomile flowers   3 parts althaea roots
> 1 part calendula flowers   1 part linden flowers
> 1 part flax seeds

Prepare and take as above.

Acute Gastritis

The following complex recipes are used in Russia to help people suffering from acute gastritis, the clinical term for stomach inflammation. It is often accompanied by severe pain, abdominal tenderness, nausea, and vomiting. Anorexia and prostration may accompany the symptoms. The formulas included here should be taken as soon as possible after symptoms appear.

ACUTE GASTRITIS RECIPE 1

1 part St. Johnswort	2 parts chamomile flowers
2 parts plantain leaves	1 part calendula flowers
1 part peppermint leaves	

Add 1 cup (250 ml) of boiling water to 1 teaspoon (5 g) of herbal mixture. Cover and steep for 30 minutes. Strain. Take $^1/_3$ cup (80 ml) every hour. Three to 4 cups (750 ml to 1 liter) can be taken during the course of the day.

In some patients, the first several doses may cause vomiting. In addition, the patient may experience strong bowel movements, which will subside after the first 6 hours. Repeated doses of the formula should cause no adverse side effects after the first few hours.

As a rule, the patient abstains from food during the first day of treatment. Some light food, such as milk or rice porridge, is permitted during the second day. Additional foods can be added gradually over 3 to 4 days until diet is normalized.

ACUTE GASTRITIS RECIPE 2

1 part St. Johnswort	2 parts yarrow
4 parts chamomile flowers	

Prepare as above. Take $^1/_2$ cup (125 ml) 4 to 5 times daily.

Chronic Gastritis

Chronic gastritis is one of the most common digestive disorders. Symptoms include an uncomfortable feeling of fullness after a small meal, mild nausea and anorexia, a bad taste in the mouth, and mild or acute pain in the region over the pit of the stomach. In about two-thirds of the cases, it is followed by inflammation of the gall bladder, colitis, or diseases of the liver.

Many Russian healers take a holistic approach to treating chronic gastritis. In addition to using complex herbal recipes, some herbalists recommend special diets involving five to six small meals a day instead of three larger ones. They stress that it is important that the patient strive to eliminate the basic causes of the problem rather than merely treat the symptoms. If not, whatever treatments are used—whether allopathic or herbal or both—will not be successful.

The following recipes are used in Russia to treat chronic gastritis alone and chronic gastritis accompanied by other symptoms like diarrhea or constipation. Some recipes are also designed to address the various causes of chronic gastritis, such as low or excess stomach acidity.

CHRONIC GASTRITIS RECIPE 1

4 parts peppermint leaves   1 part yarrow
3 parts chamomile flowers

Add 1 cup (250 ml) of boiling water to 1 teaspoon (5 g) of herbal mixture. Cover and steep for 6 hours. Strain. Take ¹/₂ cup (125 ml) for 2 to 4 weeks 3 times a day before meals. Continuing to take this formula after symptoms subside will help prevent a relapse.

CHRONIC GASTRITIS RECIPE 2

2 parts plantain leaves   1 part fennel seeds
2 parts chamomile flowers   1 part peppermint leaves

Prepare and take as above. This recipe is also taken after symptoms subside to prevent a relapse.

CHRONIC GASTRITIS RECIPE 3

2 parts peppermint leaves   1 part yarrow
1 part dill seeds   1 part restharrow roots

Add 1¹/₂ teaspoons (7 g) of herbal mixture to 1 cup (250 ml) of cold water. Cover and let stand for 8 hours. Heat to boiling, then reduce heat and gently simmer for 5 minutes. Allow to cool to room temperature. Strain. Take ¹/₂ cup (125 ml) 2 to 3 times a day before meals if chronic gastritis is followed by constipation. A single course of treatment lasts from 5 to 7 days or until bowel movements are normalized.

CHRONIC GASTRITIS RECIPE 4

1 part restharrow roots	1 part plantain leaves
2 parts marjoram	3 parts chamomile flowers
1 part nettle leaves	

Add 1¹/₂ teaspoons (7 g) of herbal mixture to 1 cup (250 ml) of water. Heat on a low flame to boiling and continue to boil for 10 minutes. Filter. Take ¹/₃ cup (80 ml) 3 times a day after meals. Like the previous formula, this also aids in normalizing bowel function.

CHRONIC GASTRITIS RECIPE 5

2 parts plantain leaves	1 part milfoil leaves
2 parts thyme	1 part licorice roots
3 parts peppermint leaves	

Add 1 cup (250 ml) of boiling water to 1 teaspoon (5 g) of herbal mixture. Cover and steep for 30 minutes. Filter. Take ¹/₂ cup (125 ml) 4 times daily in cases when chronic gastritis is accompanied by dyskinesia (impairment of intestinal movement) followed by persistent constipation.

CHRONIC GASTRITIS RECIPE 6

4 parts chamomile flowers	1 part licorice roots
1 part peppermint leaves	2 parts cudweed herb

Prepare as above. Take 1 cup (250 ml) before breakfast and 1 cup before dinner. This complex formula is used for the same symptoms as the previous recipe.

CHRONIC GASTRITIS RECIPE 7

4 parts peppermint leaves	2 parts chamomile flowers
3 parts everlasting	2 parts dill seeds
3 parts yarrow	

Place 1 tablespoon (15 g) of herbal mix in a thermos bottle and add 3 cups (750 ml) of boiling water. Seal and allow to stand for 10 to 12 hours. Take 1 cup (250 ml) upon rising in the morning, 1 cup before lunch, and 1 cup before dinner. This recipe is recommended primarily for those suffering from acute gastritis due to low stomach acidity.

CHRONIC GASTRITIS RECIPE 8

1 part althaea roots	1 part licorice roots
1 part chamomile flowers	1 part fennel seeds

Pour 1 cup (250 ml) of boiling water into a thermos containing 1 teaspoon (5 g) of herbal mixture. Prepare as above. Take 1 cup (250 ml) before dinner. This formula is used to treat the same symptoms as the previous recipe.

CHRONIC GASTRITIS RECIPE 9

1 part plantain leaves	2 parts buckbean leaves
1 part rowanberries	

Prepare as above. Take 1/3 cup (80 ml) 3 times daily before meals for similar diagnosis.

CHRONIC GASTRITIS RECIPE 10

4 parts chamomile flowers	3 parts yarrow
3 parts St. Johnswort	

Prepare as above. Take 1/3 cup (80 ml) 3 times daily before meals for chronic gastritis due to excess stomach acidity.

CHRONIC GASTRITIS RECIPE 11

4 parts St. Johnswort	2 parts calendula flowers
1 part linden flowers	

Prepare and take as above for chronic gastritis with normal stomach acid secretions.

CHRONIC GASTRITIS RECIPE 12

1 part cinquefoil roots	2 parts bilberries
1 part thyme seeds	1 part strawflower flowers
3 parts sage leaves	

Add 1 teaspoon (5 g) of herbal mixture to 1 cup (250 ml) of boiling water. Continue to boil gently for 5 minutes. Pour into a thermos, close, and allow to stand for 3 to 4 hours. Take 1/3 cup (80 ml) 3 times a day before meals for chronic gastritis accompanied by dyskinesia with diarrhea.

CHRONIC GASTRITIS RECIPE 13

| 1 part strawflower flowers | 5 parts sage leaves |
| 1 part thyme seeds | 2 parts cinquefoil roots |

Add 1 cup (250 ml) of boiling hot water to 1 tablespoon (15 g) of herbal mixture. Cover and steep for 1 hour. Filter. Take $^1/_3$ cup (80 ml) 3 times a day before meals. This recipe is designed to treat the same symptoms as the previous formula.

CHRONIC GASTRITIS RECIPE 14

4 parts chamomile flowers	1 part peppermint leaves
2 parts plantain leaves	1 part yarrow
2 parts St. Johnswort	

Add 1 teaspoon (5 g) of herbal mixture to 1 cup (250 ml) of cold water. Cover and let stand for 8 hours. Heat to boiling, then reduce heat and simmer gently for 5 minutes. Allow to cool to room temperature. Take $^1/_2$ cup (125 ml) before breakfast and another $^1/_2$ cup (125 ml) before dinner. This recipe can be used alone or may be added to the basic recipes (Chronic Gastritis 1 and 2) for chronic gastritis if accompanied by dyskinesia of the ducts which bring bile from the liver to the hepatic duct.

CHRONIC GASTRITIS RECIPE 15

| 4 parts chamomile flowers | 1 part St. Johnswort |
| 2 parts plantain leaves | 1 part yarrow |

Add 1 tablespoon (15 g) of herb mixture to 1 cup (250 ml) of water. Heat to boiling, then reduce heat and simmer gently for 5 minutes. Pour into a thermos bottle, close, and allow to stand for 6 hours. Filter. Take $^1/_2$ cup (125 ml) 4 times a day 1 hour after mealtimes. This recipe is recommended for those suffering from chronic gastritis due to low stomach acidity accompanied by diarrhea and distension caused by abdominal or intestinal gas.

Stomach and Duodenal Ulcers

A stomach ulcer is an open sore on the mucous membrane of the stomach, while a duodenal ulcer is found on the mucosa of the duodenum. The terms *peptic ulcer* and *gastric ulcer* refer to both types of ulcer. Ulcers are believed to be caused by the action of gastric juice, although recent findings point to a viral component as well. Chronic stress due to nervous disorders, infections, or prolonged steroid therapy are believed to play a role in triggering symptoms of ulcer in some individuals.

Approximately 50 percent of all allopathic medications used to treat ulcer in Russia are derived from herbs. Since many traditional ulcer medications can produce adverse side effects, herbal preparations are often recommended to ameliorate such reactions. As with other diseases, herbalists stress the importance of being under the care of a physician, especially if the patient experiences a relapse. When left untreated, gastric ulcers can produce bleeding, a life-threatening condition that may require emergency surgery.

Generally speaking, the same herbal formulas used to treat chronic gastritis (when accompanied by excess stomach acid secretions) can be used for treating stomach or duodenal ulcers. However, the following recipes have been designed specifically to treat this problem.

Ulcer Recipe 1

1 part plantain leaves   2 parts everlasting
2 parts chamomile flowers   1 part yarrow

Pour 1 cup (250 ml) of water into a pot and add 1 tablespoon (15 g) of herbal mixture. Heat to boiling, then reduce heat and simmer for 5 minutes. Pour into a thermos, close, and allow to steep for 6 hours. Take ½ cup (125 ml) 3 times daily before meals.

Ulcer Recipe 2

1 part dill seeds   2 parts chamomile flowers
1 part althaea roots   1 part licorice roots

Prepare as above. Take ⅓ cup (80 ml) 4 times a day after meals.

Ulcer Recipe 3

1 part plantain leaves   1 part yarrow
2 parts chamomile flowers   1 part licorice roots

Prepare and take as above.

In the event of a relapse involving stomach pain and heartburn, the following complex recipes are often prescribed:

ULCER RECIPE 4

1 part chamomile flowers   3 parts coltsfoot
2 parts calendula flowers

Prepare and take as above.

ULCER RECIPE 5

1 part licorice roots   1 part fennel seeds
1 part chamomile flowers   1 part St. Johnswort

Prepare and take as above.

ULCER RECIPE 6

1 part everlasting   1 part peppermint leaves
1 part chamomile flowers   1 part calendula flowers
1 part St. Johnswort

Prepare and take as above.

ULCER RECIPE 7

1 part plantain leaves   2 parts peppermint leaves
1 part licorice roots   1 part valerian roots
1 part chamomile flowers   2 parts hawthorn flowers

Add $1^{1}/_{2}$ teaspoons (7 g) of herbal mixture to a pot containing 1 cup (250 ml) of boiling water. Reduce heat and simmer for 10 to 15 seconds. Pour into a thermos, close, and allow to stand for 4 hours. Take $^{1}/_{4}$ cup (60 ml) 3 times a day before meals. This formula is prescribed to relieve pain in the heart area exacerbated by ulcer symptoms.

ULCER RECIPE 8

1 part St. Johnswort   1 part nettle leaves
1 part calendula flowers   1 part peppermint leaves
2 parts everlasting

Prepare as above. Take ¼ cup (60 ml) 4 times daily before meals. This recipe is generally recommended for the symptoms of an ulcer and should be taken for up to 3 weeks.

ULCER RECIPE 9

1 part everlasting   1 part rose hips
1 part plantain leaves

Prepare and take as above. This recipe is recommended during the period of scar formation from the fourth to sixth week after the onset of symptoms.

ULCER RECIPE 10

1 part chamomile flowers   3 parts St. Johnswort
1 part tormentil roots

Prepare and use as above, but use 1 tablespoon (15 g) of herbal mixture and boil for 5 minutes. Take ¼ cup 4 times daily before meals. This recipe is recommended for bleeding ulcers; however, herbalists recommend that at any onset of bleeding a physician should be consulted immediately.

Intestinal Disorders

There is a wide range of intestinal diseases. Enterocolitis involves inflammation of the intestines and the colon, whereas colitis involves only inflammation of the colon. These diseases are not to be taken lightly. Enterocolitis, for example, can produce shock and upset the electrolyte balance of the body (electrolytes are vital for conducting energy within the body). It requires immediate medical treatment, which usually includes antibiotics.

Before any herbal treatments are given, Russian healers stress the importance of a competent medical diagnosis. Some intestinal disorders may be due to diverticulitis, spastic colon cancer, or other problems that call for specific types of medical therapy.

On the following pages, we will list some of the complex herbal recipes used in Russia to treat a variety of intestinal problems.

Intestinal Irritation

The following herbal recipes are used to relieve symptoms of irritation of the small intestine.

INTESTINAL IRRITATION RECIPE 1

1 part restharrow roots
2 parts chamomile flowers

1 part valerian roots
1 part peppermint leaves

Add 1 tablespoon (15 g) of herbal mixture to 1 cup (250 ml) of cold water. Cover and allow to stand for 2 hours. Bring to a boil, then reduce heat and simmer gently for 5 minutes. Pour into a thermos bottle, close, and let stand for 4 hours. Strain. Take ¹/₄ cup (60 ml) before breakfast and another before dinner.

INTESTINAL IRRITATION RECIPE 2

1 part chamomile flowers
1 part valerian leaves
1 part peppermint leaves

1 part fennel seeds
1 part thyme seeds

Prepare and take as above.

INTESTINAL IRRITATION RECIPE 3

1 part calendula flowers
2 parts linden flowers

1 part sage leaves
1 part birch leaves

Prepare and take as above.

INTESTINAL IRRITATION RECIPE 4

1 part fennel seeds
1 part milfoil

1 part mugwort
1 part sweet flag roots

Prepare and take as above.

Dyskinesia

The following recipes are used in cases when dyskinesia (impairment of intestinal movement) is accompanied by constipation. Russian herbalists suggest that the course of treatment stop when the symptoms cease.

DYSKINESIA RECIPE 1

> 1 part restharrow roots
> 1 part licorice roots
> 1 part althaea roots
>
> 1 part fennel seeds
> 1 part flaxseeds
>
> Prepare and take as above.

DYSKINESIA RECIPE 2

> 2 parts elecampane roots
> 2 parts licorice roots
> 1 part angelica roots
>
> 1 part valerian roots
> 3 parts buckthorn seeds
>
> Prepare and take as above.

DYSKINESIA RECIPE 3

> 1 part restharrow roots
> 2 parts angelica roots
>
> 1 part fennel seeds
>
> Grind the mixture into a powder. Take 1 level teaspoon (5 g) of the well-mixed powder 3 times a day before meals. You can also take some water to make it easier to swallow.

Enteral Syndrome

Enteral syndrome is a term Russian healers use to describe a complex medical problem involving intestinal pain (located right behind the navel) accompanied by weight loss, digestive disorders, diarrhea (4 to 6 times a day), and intestinal distension caused by excess gas, known clinically as *meteorism*. When bowel movements normalize, continue taking the recipes for 5 or 6 more days. However, herbalists suggest reducing the dosages of bilberries, cinquefoil, and bistort by two-thirds.

If bowel movements become normal but symptoms of meteorism persist, add 1 part licorice roots or 2 parts of calendula flowers to any of the recipes. You can double the amount of chamomile flowers in any recipe as well.

ENTERAL SYNDROME RECIPE 1

1 part peppermint leaves   1 part cinquefoil roots
2 parts rose hips   2 parts chamomile flowers
1 part milfoil leaves

Add 1 tablespoon (15 g) of mixture to 1 cup (250 ml) of water. Cover and let stand for 2 hours. Heat to boiling, then reduce heat and simmer for 5 minutes. Pour into a thermos bottle, close, and let stand for another 4 hours. Filter. Take ¹/₄ cup (60 ml) before breakfast and another before dinner.

ENTERAL SYNDROME RECIPE 2

1 part cinquefoil roots   2 parts bilberry leaves
3 parts bilberries   5 parts chamomile flowers

Prepare and take as above.

ENTERAL SYNDROME RECIPE 3

2 parts Iceland moss   1 part chamomile flowers
1 part cinquefoil roots   3 parts bistort roots

Prepare and take as above.

ENTERAL SYNDROME RECIPE 4

3 parts Iceland moss   5 parts chamomile flowers
2 parts bilberries   3 parts bistort roots

Prepare and take as above.

Colitis

Colitis is a painful, chronic, and debilitating disease often accompanied by diarrhea or constipation. Mucus colitis is often characterized by large quantities of mucus in the colon, with pain in the middle of the abdomen. Ulcerative colitis produces ulcers in the mucosa of the colon. Symptoms include abdominal pain, tenderness, fever, and possible hemorrhage. Stools are watery, foul-smelling, and contain mucus.

The following remedies are used by Russian herbalists to help the body recover from different types of colitis. They are often used in conjunction with traditional allopathic treatment.

The following four recipes are recommended for those suffering from colitis accompanied by frequent diarrhea.

MUCUS COLITIS RECIPE 1

3 parts cinquefoil roots   1 part peppermint leaves
2 parts bistort roots   1 part chamomile flowers

Add 1 teaspoon (5 g) of herbal mixture to 1 cup (250 ml) of water. Cover and allow to stand for 2 hours. Bring to a boil, then reduce heat and simmer gently for 5 minutes. Pour contents into a thermos, close, and let stand for 4 hours. Filter. Take 1 cup (250 ml) 3 times a day before meals.

MUCUS COLITIS RECIPE 2

1 part fennel seeds   3 parts sage leaves
1 part oak bark

Prepare and take as above.

MUCUS COLITIS RECIPE 3

1 part sweet flag roots   1 part bilberries
2 parts thyme

Prepare as above. Take a total of 1 cup (250 ml) a day, sipping a little at a time.

MUCUS COLITIS RECIPE 4

1 part chamomile flowers   1 part bilberries
1 part plantain leaves   1 part bistort root

Prepare as above. Take 1 cup (250 ml) 3 times a day before meals.

The following three recipes are recommended for those suffering from colitis accompanied by constipation.

MUCUS COLITIS RECIPE 5

1 part restharrow roots	1 part buckbean leaves
1 part nettle leaves	

Add 1 teaspoon (5 g) of herbal mixture to 1 cup (250 ml) of water. Bring to a boil, then reduce heat and simmer gently for 5 minutes. Cover and let stand for a half hour. Filter. Take $^1/_2$ cup (125 ml) before bedtime.

MUCUS COLITIS RECIPE 6

3 parts restharrow roots	2 parts nettle leaves
1 part yarrow leaves	

Prepare and take as above.

MUCUS COLITIS RECIPE 7

3 parts restharrow roots	1 part aniseed
1 part buckbean leaves	3 parts buckthorn seeds
2 parts thyme seeds	

Prepare and take as above.

MUCUS COLITIS RECIPE 8

1 part sage leaves	1 part restharrow roots
1 part nettle leaves	1 part buckthorn seeds

Prepare and take as above.

The following recipes are used for bloody stools, symptomatic of bleeding of the colon mucosa.

ULCERATIVE COLITIS RECIPE 1

1 part chamomile flowers	2 parts rose hips
1 part yarrow leaves	1 part plantain leaves
1 part nettle leaves	

Prepare and take as in Mucus Colitis Recipe 1.

Ulcerative Colitis Recipe 2

5 parts chamomile flowers	1 part bistort roots
2 parts peppermint leaves	1 part yarrow leaves
3 parts St. Johnswort	3 parts nettle leaves

Prepare and take as in Mucus Colitis Recipe 1.

Stomach and Intestinal Bleeding

Bleeding can be caused by a number of diseases, including colitis, ulcers, and hemorrhoids, and can be very serious. In such cases, a physician should be called immediately for diagnosis and treatment. As with other health problems, Russian healers often use a combination of allopathic medications with herbal remedies.

As a rule, herbal treatment works more slowly than many modern drugs. In emergency situations such as hemorraging, allopathic medications are usually more appropriate. However if the problem is not an emergency, or if treatment is to take place over a longer period of time, herbs may be preferable to pharmaceuticals.

The following recipes are designed to complement traditional medical treatment for bleeding of the mucous layers of the stomach and the intestines.

Stomach Bleeding Recipe 1

1 part St. Johnswort	2 parts licorice roots
2 parts yarrow leaves	1 part barberry bark

Add 1 tablespoon (15 g) of herbal mixture to 1 cup (250 ml) of boiling water. Turn off heat, cover, and steep for 2 hours. Reheat to boiling, then reduce heat and simmer for a few seconds. Pour into a thermos bottle, close, and steep for 4 hours. Strain. Take ¹/₂ cup (125 ml) 3 times daily before meals.

Stomach Bleeding Recipe 2

4 parts chamomile flowers	1 part peppermint leaves
1 part yarrow leaves	2 parts bistort leaves
2 parts oak bark	

Prepare and take as above.

INTESTINAL BLEEDING RECIPE 1

1 part peppermint leaves
1 part plantain leaves
2 parts chamomile flowers

3 parts tormentil roots
1 part bilberry leaves
1 part oak bark

Prepare and take as above.

INTESTINAL BLEEDING RECIPE 2

2 parts coltsfoot leaves
1 part chamomile flowers
1 part birch leaves

1 part nettle leaves
1 part marjoram

Prepare as above. Take ¹/₃ cup (80 ml) 3 times a day before meals.
This recipe is recommended for patients who cough up blood.

Poor Appetite

Appetizers are not only the dishes we eat in a restaurant before we have the
main dish but also include any herbs or formulas that stimulate the desire
to eat. The following formulas are excellent appetizers, which can be used
for anyone who wishes to increase their desire for food due to depression,
physical illness, or chemotherapy.

APPETIZER RECIPE 1

4 parts mugwort
1 part yarrow leaves

Add 1 cup (250 ml) of boiling water to 1 tablespoon (15 g) of
herbal mixture. Cover and steep for 20 minutes. Take 1 to 2
tablespoons (15 to 30 g) 10 to 15 minutes before mealtimes.

APPETIZER RECIPE 2

1 part mugwort
1 part buckbean leaves

1 part thyme seeds

Prepare as above. Take 1 tablespoon (15 g) 3 to 4 times a day, 20
minutes before meals.

APPETIZER RECIPE 3

> 1 part mugwort   1 part dandelion roots
> 1 part yarrow leaves
>
> Prepare and take as above.

Diabetes Mellitus

Diabetes mellitus is a chronic and incurable metabolic disorder in which the pancreas is unable to produce sufficient quantities of insulin, a hormone necessary for the metabolism of blood sugar and the maintenance of proper blood sugar levels. Diabetes affects an increasingly large proportion of adults in North America. Symptoms include high blood sugar levels, sugar in the urine, and excessive thirst. When severe, diabetes produces nausea, weakness, intoxication, coma, and even death. Diabetics are often susceptible to a wide range of additional health problems, including bedsores, infections, cardiovascular disorders, and gangrene.

No one is sure of the cause of diabetes, although dietary factors, including high intake of sugar, may be involved. Doctors recommend a carefully supervised dietary program including a well-balanced and sugar-free diet and regular exercise; weight loss is a primary goal of treatment for obese patients in particular. If dietary management does not raise insulin levels, insulin injections are then prescribed. Although there is presently no cure for diabetes, it can often be managed by the patient under a doctor's close supervision.

In Russia, a number of herbs mentioned in this book are used to help manage diabetes. In addition, kidney beans—an unlikely but widely available food—are often used to help treat diabetes in Russia. They are important ingredients in a number of complex herbal recipes for diabetics as well as a regular part of the diet. These recipes have been found to be especially useful in milder cases of the disease or in its early stages.

DIABETES RECIPE 1

> 1 part peppermint leaves   1 part flaxseeds
> 1 part kidney beans   1 part bilberries
>   (cooked, mashed)
>
> Add 1 tablespoon (15 g) of mixture to 1 cup (250 ml) of boiling water. Cover and steep for 45 minutes. Strain. Take 1 cup (250 ml) 3 times daily before meals.

DIABETES RECIPE 2

1 part elecampane roots   3 parts rose hips
1 part St. Johnswort   3 parts bilberry leaves
1 part horsetail

Prepare as above. Take ¹/₂ cup (125 ml) 3 times daily before meals.

DIABETES RECIPE 3

1 part dandelion roots   1 part bilberry leaves
1 part kidney beans   1 part nettle leaves
   (cooked, mashed)
1 part barberry

Prepare and take as above.

DIABETES RECIPE 4

1 part kidney beans   1 part bilberry leaves
   (cooked, mashed)
1 part burdock roots

Add 1 tablespoon (15 g) of mixture to 2 cups (500 ml) of cold water. Cover and let stand for 2 hours. Heat to boiling, then reduce heat and simmer for 5 minutes. Pour into a thermos, close, and steep for 4 hours. Take ¹/₂ cup (125 ml) 5 times daily, both before and between meals.

THE LIVER AND
GALLBLADDER

꒰◦ᰔ.ᰔ◦꒱

The Liver

To most people, the liver is an inert mass located in the middle of the diaphragm. In fact, the liver, whose major task is to purify the blood, is the body's largest internal organ. It contains 350 billion specialized cells and performs over five hundred different functions. They include assimilating and storing food products that have been digested in the intestines, detoxifying the body, and secreting bile, which is necessary for the digestion of fats. It also stores many of the nutrients we need for survival, including carbohydrates, fat, protein, vitamins, and minerals. Among the early Babylonians and the Greeks, the liver was considered to be the abode of the human soul.

Russian healers have discovered that complex herbal recipes can support the liver and do much to help the body heal itself of a number of liver diseases.

Chronic Hepatitis

Hepatitis is a clinical term for inflammation of the liver, a serious disease that can be produced by a virus or toxin. Symptoms include jaundice, liver enlargement, and fever. Chronic hepatitis can last from six months to several years. There are a number of different types of hepatitis, which all require the care of a medical doctor. For chronic hepatitis a normal course of herbal treatment lasts from five to six months. This is followed by a two-month break. Another course is then recommended, followed by another break. Because liver healing is often slow, this cycle is usually continued for two to three years. The following recipes are used in Russia to provide healing support to the liver affected by all varieties of the disease.

HEPATITIS RECIPE 1

1 part peppermint leaves   1 part fennel seeds
1 part strawflower flowers   1 part yarrow

Add 1$^{1}/_{2}$ teaspoons (7 g) of herbal mixture to a pot containing 1 cup (250 ml) of boiling water. Reduce heat and simmer for 5 minutes. Pour into a thermos, close, and steep for 4 hours. Strain. Take $^{1}/_{2}$ cup (125 ml) 3 times a day before meals.

HEPATITIS RECIPE 2

2 parts strawflower flowers   2 parts birch leaves
1 part nettle leaves   1 part St. Johnswort
1 part rose hips

Prepare and take as above.

After healing has taken place, herbalists recommend a preventive course of herbal therapy for two to three months a year, especially in the spring or autumn when it is believed that people are most susceptible to a relapse. The following recipes are among the most popular.

HEPATITIS PREVENTIVE RECIPE 1

1 part chamomile flowers   1 part St. Johnswort
1 part licorice roots   1 part birch leaves
2 parts peppermint leaves

Prepare and take as above.

HEPATITIS PREVENTIVE RECIPE 2

1 part horsetail herb   1 part sage
1 part calendula flowers   1 part rose hips
1 part yarrow

Prepare and take as above.

Hepatitis Preventive Recipe 3

2 parts licorice roots
1 part celandine herb
1 part marjoram

2 parts chamomile flowers
2 parts peppermint leaves

Prepare and take as above.

Hepatitis Preventive Recipe 4

2 parts dandelion roots
2 parts buckbean leaves
2 parts horsetail

1 part thyme seeds
1 part rose hips

Prepare and take as above.

Cirrhosis of the Liver

Cirrhosis is a very serious chronic disease that is often brought on by alcoholism combined with impaired nutrition, although other causes may be responsible, like poisoning. At first, the liver enlarges, then later becomes shrunken and atrophied. The disease involves degenerative changes in liver cells and the formation of dense connective tissue, which impairs liver function. It is often fatal. The following recipes have long been used in Russia to help restore liver function affected by cirrhosis.

Cirrhosis Recipe 1

1 part rose hips
2 parts strawflower flowers

1 part nettle leaves

Add $1^1/_2$ teaspoons (7 g) of herbal mixture to a pot containing 1 cup (250 ml) of boiling water. Reduce heat and simmer for 5 minutes. Pour into a thermos, close, and allow to stand for 4 hours. Filter. Take 1 cup (250 ml) over the course of the day, sipping a little at a time.

Cirrhosis Recipe 2

1 part thyme seeds
1 part calendula flowers
1 part chamomile flowers

1 part licorice roots
1 part rose hips

Prepare as above. Take $^1/_2$ cup (125 ml) before breakfast and another before dinner.

CIRRHOSIS RECIPE 3

2 parts rose hips
1 part nettle leaves
3 parts carrot root (grated)

1 part rowanberries
2 parts calendula flowers

Prepare as above. Take ½ cup (125 ml) 3 times a day with meals.

The Gallbladder

The primary function of the gallbladder is to hold bile from the liver before discharging it into the duodenum. Bile is necessary for the digestion of fats, and it is also a natural purgative and antiseptic. Gallstones are formed in the gallbladder or bile ducts when the free flow of bile is impeded in the gallbladder. Their presence does not cause pain until the bladder becomes inflamed. Once it does, pain can be extreme.

Over generations, Russian herbalists have developed a number of fine herbal formulas for treating some of the most common problems affecting the gallbladder and bile ducts. As with other treatments, those listed here are often used as complements to traditional medical therapy.

Chronic Cholecystitis

Cholecystitis is a clinical term for inflammation of the gallbladder. While acute cholecystitis is almost always caused by gallstones, chronic cholecystitis may occur with or without them.

Herbal treatment is recommended after detailed examination by a physician to insure that there are no stones present or that the patient's complaints are not due to other factors.

CHRONIC CHOLECYSTITIS RECIPE 1

1 part St. Johnswort
1 part restharrow
4 parts strawflower flowers

2 parts chamomile flowers
1 part juniper berries

Add 1 tablespoon (15 g) of herbal mixture to 1 cup (250 ml) of cold water. Cover and let stand for 2 hours. Heat to boiling, then reduce heat and simmer for 2 to 3 minutes. Pour into a thermos, close, and allow to stand for 8 hours. Strain. Take ½ cup (125 ml) 4 times a day 1 hour after meals.

Chronic Cholecystitis Recipe 2

1 part sweet flag roots   1 part calendula flowers
1 part strawflower flowers

Prepare as above. Take ¹/₄ cup (60 ml) 4 times daily.

Chronic Cholecystitis Recipe 3

2 parts peppermint leaves   1 part St. Johnswort
1 part valerian roots   1 part buckbean leaves

Add 1 cup (250 ml) of boiling water to 1 tablespoon (15 g) of herbal mixture. Cover and steep for 30 minutes. Filter. Take ¹/₂ cup (125 ml) twice a day before meals.

Gallstones (Cholelithiasis)

Cholelithiasis describes the formation of gallstones. At the present time, some allopathic medications are used to help dissolve gallstones, but if they are unsuccessful, surgery may be necessary.

Russian herbal therapy has never been highly effective in dissolving gallstones. Although Russian herbalists have had some success in remedies that assist in passing stones, the treatments often can take months, causing considerable discomfort to the patient. Today, most patients prefer surgery, which is a fast and relatively safe procedure.

Having said this, we are including some old recipes that may be used as preventive measures for individuals who are prone to gallstones. They also may be useful for patients whose stones are in the very beginning of formation.

Gallstone Recipe 1

3 parts strawflower flowers   3 parts milfoil
2 parts restharrow roots

Add 1 cup (250 ml) of boiling water to 1 teaspoon (5 g) of herbal mixture. Cover and steep for 20 minutes. Strain. Take 1 cup (250 ml) daily before dinner.

GALLSTONE RECIPE 2

> 1 part peppermint leaves   1 part restharrow roots
> 1 part mugwort   1 part dandelion roots
> 1 part strawflower flowers
>
> Prepare and take as above.

GALLSTONE RECIPE 3

> 2 parts St. Johnswort   4 parts strawflower flowers
> 1 part chamomile flowers   1 part restharrow roots
>
> Prepare and take as above.

THE KIDNEYS AND
URINARY TRACT

❧❀❧

The kidneys are very important to us. They produce and excrete urine and help regulate the water, electrolytes, and acids in the blood.

On the following pages, we will examine some diseases that affect the kidneys and the urinary tract and find out which Russian complex herbal formulas can help the body to heal them.

Glomerulonephritis

Nephritis is a clinical term that describes inflammation of the kidneys. Glomerulonephritis is a type of nephritis affecting the glomeruli, which are small structures within the kidney made up of clusters of capillaries surrounded by a thin membrane and are involved in the production of urine.

Acute Glomerulonephritis

Acute glomerulonephritis is usually treated with bed rest, salt-free diets, and allopathic medications such as antibiotics. The existing research regarding herbal recipes shows that while treatment is often slow, the herbal formulas do not produce adverse side effects like some pharmaceutical preparations. For this reason, Russian physicians often prefer to use both traditional medications and complex herbal formulas.

Herbalists advise that the following formulas should not be taken in conjunction with other herbal preparations containing horsetail, birch, or juniper berries. Kidney problems should be diagnosed by a competent physician.

ACUTE GLOMERULONEPHRITIS RECIPE 1

3 parts lemon balm   1 part marjoram
1 part calendula flowers   2 parts motherwort

Add 1 tablespoon (15 g) of herbal mixture to 1 cup (250 ml) of water. Heat to boiling, then reduce heat and simmer gently for 5 minutes. Pour into a thermos, close, and let stand for 4 hours. Filter. Take $^1/_4$ cup (60 ml) 4 times daily before mealtimes. A small amount of honey may be added if desired.

ACUTE GLOMERULONEPHRITIS RECIPE 2

1 part calendula flowers   1 part nettle leaves
1 part motherwort

Prepare and take as above.

ACUTE GLOMERULONEPHRITIS RECIPE 3

1 part St. Johnswort herb   1 part arnica flowers
1 part nettle leaves   1 part calendula flowers

Prepare and take as above. This recipe is recommended for patients whose kidney inflammation is accompanied by bleeding.

Chronic Glomerulonephritis

Chronic glomerulonephritis can take several forms, known in medical literature as latent, hypertonic, endemic, and mixed. The following herbal recipes complement traditional medical therapy in Russia, depending on the physician's diagnosis.

CHRONIC GLOMERULONEPHRITIS RECIPE 1

1 part St. Johnswort   2 parts calendula flowers
1 part pansy   1 part lemon balm leaves

Prepare as described in the recipes above. Take $^1/_4$ cup (60 ml) 3 times a day. This recipe is recommended for patients suffering from the latent form of this disease.

CHRONIC GLOMERULONEPHRITIS RECIPE 2

1 part Iceland moss	1 part calendula flowers
2 parts lemon balm leaves	1 part parsley seeds
2 parts linden flowers	

Add 1½ teaspoons (7 g) of herbal mix to 1 cup (250 ml) of cold water. Cover and let stand for 2 hours. Bring to a boil, then reduce heat and simmer gently for 5 minutes. Pour into a thermos bottle and steep for 4 hours. Filter. Take ¼ cup (60 ml) 3 times a day before meals. This recipe will cause perspiration and is likely to produce both anti-inflammatory and depurative actions.

CHRONIC GLOMERULONEPHRITIS RECIPE 3

1 part elecampane roots	1 part elder flowers
2 parts St. Johnswort	1 part betony
1 part Iceland moss	

Prepare and take as above. This recipe is prescribed to improve the secretory and excretory functions of the kidneys.

CHRONIC GLOMERULONEPHRITIS RECIPE 4

1 part calendula flowers	2 parts sage
1 part shepherd's purse	1 part motherwort

Prepare and take as above. This recipe is recommended as an all-purpose remedy for this disease. After 4 weeks of use, herbalists recommend shifting to the following recipe.

CHRONIC GLOMERULONEPHRITIS RECIPE 5

1 part calendula flowers	3 parts lemon balm
1 part dill seeds	2 parts Iceland moss

Prepare and take as above for 4 weeks. After this time, repeat Chronic Glomerulonephritis Recipe 4 for another 4 weeks. Recipes 4 and 5 may be alternated in the future as needed.

Chronic Pyelonephritis

Pyelonephritis involves inflammation of the kidney substance and pelvis. After diagnosis, the physician usually recommends that the causes of this disease be addressed, such as infections, chronic tonsillitis, severe tooth decay, or boils. Although these may be minor symptoms in themselves, their secretions are carried to the kidneys, where they produce irritation and inflammation. Russian doctors also recommend a course of antibiotics along with herbs. The course of antibiotic therapy usually lasts for six to eight weeks and is then continued for eight to ten days a month. Between these times, herbal therapy is recommended.

While herbs have been successful in treating this problem, in cases of severe and chronic kidney insufficiency, the selection of herbs should be made by an expert. Special precautions should be taken with prescribing herbs such as juniper berries and horsetail and preparations made with barley, aloe vera, and celandine due to their potential to irritate the kidneys.

PYELONEPHRITIS RECIPE 1

1 part birch leaves	1 part althaea roots
1 part nettle leaves	1 part bilberry leaves
2 parts Iceland moss	

Place 1 tablespoon (15 g) of herbal mixture into a pot containing 1 cup (250 ml) of cold water. Cover and allow to stand for 2 hours. Heat to boiling, then reduce heat and simmer for a few seconds. Pour into a thermos, close, and steep for 2 hours. Strain. Take 2 tablespoons (30 g) 4 times daily after meals.

PYELONEPHRITIS RECIPE 2

2 parts pansy leaves	1 part shepherd's purse leaves
2 parts calendula flowers	2 parts birch leaves

Prepare as above. Take $1/3$ cup (80 ml) 3 times a day before meals. Herbalists recommend that this recipe be alternated with the previous recipe every 2 weeks for best results.

PYELONEPHRITIS RECIPE 3

1 part nettle leaves	3 parts pansy
2 parts yarrow	3 parts coltsfoot leaves
3 parts St. Johnswort	

Add 1 cup (250 ml) of boiling water to 1 tablespoon (15 g) of herbal mixture. Cover and steep for 4 hours. Strain. Take ¹/₂ cup (125 ml) twice a day after meals.

For some patients, this recipe is considered more effective than the previous two. If the other recipes do not produce desired results, the recommended course of treatment for this recipe lasts from 20 to 25 days. You may go back to the other recipes after that time for 2 to 3 months. After that time, you can take this recipe again if needed.

Urolithiasis

This disease involves a blockage of the urinary tract due to the formation of stones (calculi). Symptoms include impediment or stoppage of urine flow, and is often accompanied by pain. Physicians usually remove the stones with a special surgical instrument that is introduced through the urethra into the bladder and ureter.

Traditionally, Russian doctors have also treated this problem with herbs, primarily in an effort to avoid recurrences. After six to eight weeks of herbal therapy the stones and sand will begin to be excreted from the body with the urine. It is not always a painless process, but the discomfort is not extreme. While taking these herbs, patients often feel that they need to urinate even if they don't have much urine in their bladder. However, herbalists suggest that they wait until the pressure in the bladder builds, indicating that there is indeed urine present. This is believed to enable the stones to be flushed out easier. Depending on the size and the number of stones, this phase of the healing process can last from one to ten days after herbal treatment begins. In addition, doctors have long stressed an increased consumption of fresh fruit and vegetable juices, as well as a low-salt diet.

In addition to herbs, Russian herbalists often prescribe a course of hydrotherapy, especially for patients prone to relapse. They suggest a warm bath (99 to 105°F or 37 to 41°C) for half an hour two or three times a day. Herbalists also recommend drinking a cup of linden flower tea during the bath. If the patient has the urge to urinate while taking the bath, herbal healers suggest that the patient refrain from doing so until the 30-minute bath is over. While this may prove somewhat uncomfortable for the patient, herbalists believe that urinating under pressure will help the body to excrete the calculi. Although the combined herbal treatment and hydrotherapy is claimed to be very effective, patients suffering from circulatory problems should consult a physician before undergoing hydrotherapy.

Depending on the type of urolithiasis and any additional symptoms, the following complex herbal formulas are used to both prevent and treat the formation of calculi in the urinary system.

UROLITHIASIS RECIPE 1

1 part uva ursi leaves	1 part juniper berries
1 part pansy	1 part birch leaves

Add 1 tablespoon (15 g) of herbal mixture to 1 cup (250 ml) of water. Cover and let stand for 2 hours. Heat to boiling, then reduce heat and simmer for a few seconds. Pour into a thermos, close, and steep for another 2 hours. Strain. Take 1 cup 3 times a day. This and the following recipe are especially designed for patients whose stones contain phosphate and carbonate.

UROLITHIASIS RECIPE 2

2 parts burdock roots	1 part dandelion
1 part shepherd's purse	1 part pansy
1 part St. Johnswort	

Prepare and take as above.

UROLITHIASIS RECIPE 3

3 parts celandine	1 part pansy
2 parts barberry leaves	1 part nettle leaves

Prepare as above. Take 1 cup (250 ml) 3 times daily. This and the following three recipes are recommended when strong acidity is present in the urine.

UROLITHIASIS RECIPE 4

2 parts yarrow	1 part horsetail
1 part nettle leaves	1 part arnica flowers

Prepare and take as above.

UROLITHIASIS RECIPE 5

5 parts birch leaves   1 part pansy
1 part horsetail

Prepare as above. Take $\frac{1}{4}$ cup (60 ml) 4 to 5 times a day.

UROLITHIASIS RECIPE 6

1 part peppermint leaves   1 part horsetail
1 part pansy   3 parts St. Johnswort
2 parts thyme

Prepare and take as above.

THE CARDIOVASCULAR
SYSTEM

❧❧

As in North America, heart disease is a major cause of death and disability in Russia. Like their counterparts in the West, researchers there have found that the heart is not an island unto itself that simply pumps blood throughout the body. It is part of a complex interplay of nerves, organs, and tissues that make up the entire body. The heart and cardiovascular system, which includes veins and arteries, responds to the kinds of foods we eat, the types of exercise we perform, and the ever-changing state of our emotions.

There are several major diseases that affect the heart and the rest of the cardiovascular system, including atherosclerosis, ischemic heart disease, and cardiac arrhythmia. With proper medical care and an ongoing program of proper diet, aerobic exercise, and stress management, cardiovascular disease can often be reversed or controlled. Yet, since many heart-related diseases can be life threatening, diagnosis and treatment should involve the care of a qualified health professional, usually a cardiologist.

As in other areas of health care, most Russian doctors use traditional allopathic therapy (including medications and surgery) for patients suffering from heart and cardiovascular disease. However, they often prescribe a variety of herbal treatments in addition to help prevent the onset of cardiovascular disease and to help the patient recover from a disease that has already been diagnosed.

Arteriosclerosis

Arteriosclerosis is a disease in which fatty deposits accumulate on the walls of blood vessels that carry blood to the heart. Arteriosclerosis is thought to be due to a metabolic defect involving lipids (fats) and lipoproteins and is especially prevalent among sedentary individuals who consume large amounts of saturated fat in their diets. It is the most common cause of coronary occlusion, which leads to heart attack.

Russian researchers have found that herbal therapy can be very useful for helping prevent arteriosclerosis and to improve lipid metabolism in the body, although they stress that patients with this disease should be monitored regularly by a qualified health-care professional. Some Russian physicians actually use chemically purified herbal extracts as medications that are injected into the patient. We will not be describing these preparations here because they require complex preparation in the laboratory and are not readily available to the majority of readers. In addition, they should always be administered by a licensed medical doctor.

The primary herbs used by Russian herbalists to prevent and treat arteriosclerosis are familiar to many of us. They include onion, garlic, motherwort herb, valerian roots, horsetail herb, and mint. Auxiliary herbs include (but are not limited to) lemon balm, pheasant's eye, raspberries, wild marjoram, and cudweed. Russian herbalists recommend eating generous amounts of onions, garlic, and raspberries (when in season) in addition to taking one of the complex recipes listed. Odor-controlled garlic supplements may be taken if eating several cloves of fresh garlic daily is not desired.

How do you know which complex recipe is right for you? Usually it takes two or even three tries to choose a recipe that will be the most effective for a particular situation. When the right one is found, herbalists suggest taking the recipe for four to six months over the course of a year, which is considered the optimum period of time that the recipe will be effective. Other herbalists recommend two courses of four months each. However, if symptoms return due to a factor like increased stress, the course should be renewed for another two months.

ARTERIOSCLEROSIS RECIPE 1

2 parts motherwort   1 part chamomile flowers
1 part valerian roots

Add 1 cup (250 ml) of boiling water to 1 teaspoon (5 g) of the herbal mixture. Cover and let stand for 30 minutes. Take $^1/_2$ cup (125 ml) 3 times a day 1 hour before meals.

ARTERIOSCLEROSIS RECIPE 2

2 parts lemon balm	1 part horsetail herb
1 part pheasant's eye	1 part cudweed herb

Prepare as above. Take ¹/₄ cup (60 ml) 3 times a day.

ARTERIOSCLEROSIS RECIPE 3

2 parts valerian root	1 part wild marjoram
2 parts lemon balm	1 part pheasant's eye

Prepare as above. Take ¹/₂ cup (125 ml) 3 times daily.

ARTERIOSCLEROSIS RECIPE 4

1 part motherwort	1 part peppermint
1 part valerian roots	

Prepare as above, but steep for 15 minutes. Take ¹/₃ cup (80 ml) 4 times a day.

Ischemic Heart Disease (IHD)

Ischemic heart disease (IHD) is defined as a local or temporary anemia due to obstruction of an artery. IHD can be fatal and involve related diseases like myocarditis (inflammation of the heart muscle), angina pectoris (heart pain due to insufficient blood flow to the heart), tachycardia (abnormal quickening of heart rhythm), and cardiac or myocardial infarction, or heart attack. When such an infarction occurs, a blocked artery prevents the blood supply from reaching the heart. As a result, the heart muscle (or parts of the muscle) can die, often with fatal consequences for the victim. Heart attack is presently the leading cause of death in the United States and most other industrialized nations.

In most cases, the same herbs used to treat arteriosclerosis are used for both the prevention and treatment of IHD. However arnica flowers and hawthorn berries are often added to the list of primary herbs. Some herbalists include licorice root, garden thyme herb, milfoil herb, and elecampane root as auxiliary herbs for IHD. Some of the most common complex recipes used in Russia include the following.

IHD Recipe 1

> 1 part valerian roots   1 part licorice roots
> 1 part yarrow leaves   1 part motherwort

Pour 1 cup (250 ml) of cold water over 1½ teaspoons (7 g) of herbal mixture. Cover and let stand for 4 hours. Heat to boiling, and continue to boil for a few seconds. Cover again and steep for 1 additional hour. Strain. Take ½ cup (125 ml) 4 to 5 times a day.

IHD Recipe 2

> 4 parts hawthorn berries   2 parts lemon balm
> 4 parts valerian roots   1 part thyme

Add 1 cup (250 ml) of boiling water to 1 teaspoon (5 g) of herbal mixture. Cover and steep for 30 minutes. Strain. Take ¼ cup (60 ml) 4 times daily.

IHD Recipe 3

> 1 part hawthorn flowers   2 parts peppermint
>   and berries   1 part elecampane

Prepare as in IHD Recipe 1. Take ¼ cup (60 ml) 4 times a day.

IHD Recipe 4

> 2 parts hawthorn berries   1 part licorice roots
> 2 parts motherwort

Add 1 cup (250 ml) of boiling water to 1 tablespoon (15 g) of herbal mixture. Steep for 10 minutes and strain. Take ½ cup (125 ml) 3 to 4 times a day 30 minutes before mealtimes.

Myocardosis

Myocardosis is a form of ischemic heart disease that involves degeneration of the heart muscle. It is often caused by an infarct or heart attack that resulted in a reduction or cessation of the blood supply to the heart muscle. Physicians stress that people who have experienced a heart attack should strive to eliminate many of its original causes, such as smoking, high intake of dietary fat, inadequate exercise, and poor response to emotional stress. In addition, postattack evaluations by a physician are invaluable for helping the patient avoid another attack in the future.

Russian herbalists prescribe many of the same herbs they use for other ischemic diseases. However they tend to be more careful when prescribing herbs for myocardosis because this disease is often accompanied by other health problems that need to be addressed as well. These additional symptoms may call for adding or removing an herb from the complex formula to make it more effective for the patient.

For some individuals, myocardosis may be accompanied by chronic constipation, which calls for the following complex recipes.

MYOCARDOSIS AND CONSTIPATION RECIPE 1

| 2 parts thyme | 1 part yarrow leaves |
| 1 part nettle | |

Add 1 cup (250 ml) of boiling water to 1 tablespoon (15 g) of herbal mixture. Steep for 10 minutes and strain. Take $^1/_2$ cup (125 ml) twice a day, early in the morning and after dinner.

MYOCARDOSIS AND CONSTIPATION RECIPE 2

| 3 parts buckthorn berries and seeds | 1 part aniseed |
| | 1 part licorice roots |

Add 1 cup (250 ml) of boiling water to 1 tablespoon (15 g) of herbal mixture. Cover, steep for 30 minutes, and strain. Take $^1/_2$ cup (125 ml) twice a day, early in the morning and after dinner.

These two recipes are usually combined with the IHD recipes presented earlier or are used in addition to these recipes. Because some people may find this inconvenient, herbalists suggest that either of these formulas can be taken after dinner and before bedtime.

Some people suffer bouts of depression after a heart attack. This is often caused by rapid or irregular heartbeat, which can make them anxious or insecure. For these patients, the following recipe is recommended.

STENOCARDIA AND DEPRESSION RECIPE 1

2 parts motherwort
1 part valerian roots
1 part peppermint

Add 1 cup (250 ml) of boiling water to 1 teaspoon (5 g) of herbal mixture. Cover and steep for 30 minutes. Strain. Take ¹/₂ cup (125 ml) in the morning and another in the evening.

For patients who experience anxiety from heart pain due to angina, Russian herbalists recommend the following recipe.

STENOCARDIA AND HEART PAIN RECIPE 1

| 1 part chamomile flowers | 3 parts peppermint |
| 2 parts fennel seeds | 1 part valerian roots |

Add 1 cup (250 ml) of boiling water to 2 teaspoons (10 g) of herbal mixture. Cover, steep for 30 minutes, and strain. Sip from time to time throughout the day, consuming 1 cup per day total.

Many herbalists use a combination therapy for ischemic heart disease and arteriosclerosis, which includes many of the recipes mentioned above combined with diuretic recipes or using a diuretic herb in the recipes. Remember that a diuretic increases the flow of urine, removes excess water that the body's tissues may be retaining, and improves blood circulation to the kidneys. The most common herbs used as diuretics are birch, restharrow, juniper berries, uva ursi, mugwort, and horsetail.

DIURETIC RECIPE 1

| 2 parts juniper berries | 1 part birch leaves |
| 2 parts horsetail | |

Add 1 cup (250 ml) of boiling water to 1 tablespoon (15 g) of herbal mixture. Steep for 10 minutes and strain. Take 3 to 4 tablespoons (45 to 60 ml) 3 to 4 times a day before meals.

DIURETIC RECIPE 2

2 parts birch leaves   1 part horsetail
1 part restharrow

Prepare as in Diuretic Recipe 1 above. Take ¹/₃ cup (80 ml) 3 times daily before meals.

DIURETIC RECIPE 3

4 parts birch leaves and buds   3 parts dandelion roots
3 parts juniper berries

Prepare as above. Take 1 tablespoon (15 g) 4 times a day before meals.

DIURETIC RECIPE 4

2 parts uva ursi leaves   2 parts mugwort leaves
1 part juniper berries   1 part restharrow

Prepare as above. Take ¹/₂ cup (125 ml) 3 times daily before meals.

Cardiovascular Insufficiency

Cardiovascular insufficiency affects the ability of the heart to function normally, which may be caused by overexertion of the heart itself or a lack of adequate blood flow into the heart. Physical overexertion or metabolic dysfunctions involving myocardosis can affect heart function. Proper diet and regular aerobic exercise are valuable in helping prevent this problem as well as in managing its symptoms.

When treating patients with heart problems, Russian herbalists pay special attention to herbs containing glucosides, which are widely distributed in plants. Many glucosides have medicinal properties that can have specific effects on the heart. Digitalin and strophanthin, both found in lily of the valley, are two such glucosides and are ingredients in digitalis, an allopathic heart medicine.

Herbal therapy for cardiac insufficiency is not unlike that for treating ischemic heart disease. However, in treating patients with cardiac insufficiency, herbalists often add a diuretic recipe prescription to a heart recipe, such as the IHD recipes presented earlier because the diuretic herbs used in these recipes produce other effects on the body in addition to their diuretic actions. Scientists still do not know exactly how these herbs work, aside from noting that their effect on patients suffering from heart problems is quite good.

Although Russian herbalists recommend that all patients suffering from symptoms of cardiac insufficiency be under the care of a qualified medical professional, they stress the value of herbs containing glucosides for treating this health problem. However, since each human being is unique, patients should be mindful of overdosing on herbs containing glucosides, especially if the heart is weak. Diuretics are especially useful in helping regulate the glucoside level in patients using these herbs. Many Russian physicians combine traditional allopathic therapy with herbal recipes, because they find that fewer medications and smaller doses are often required.

Cardiac Arrhythmia

Cardiac arrhythmia involves irregular heartbeat caused by physiological or pathological disturbances. It usually takes two forms: tachycardia, the abnormal speeding up of heart action, and bradycardia, the abnormal slowing down of the heartbeat. These three complex recipes usually produce good results in a period of days or weeks, especially when used as adjuncts to traditional allopathic treatment. While these herbs should not cause adverse side effects, it is important that the patient be carefully monitored by a professional herbalist in addition to a qualified physician. Even if the patient reports improvement, the herbalist may decide to gradually reduce the herbal dosage in stages.

Overdosing should always be avoided, especially with valerian and motherwort. As with earlier recipes, the suggested course of treatment can continue for three consecutive months during the year. Herbalists recommend that rather than discontinue the course of treatment when symptoms disappear, the patient can reduce the dosage slightly as the course of treatment progresses. Many patients report that one course of treatment is enough. Some even experience an absence of symptoms for years. However, herbalists advise patients to avoid automatically resuming a course of herbal treatment at the first sign of renewed symptoms within a year after the initial three-month period of use.

While both can be treated by drugs and other forms of medical intervention, Russian herbalists recommend the following recipes to help patients achieve normalized heartbeat.

CARDIAC ARRHYTHMIA RECIPE 1

1 part peppermint
1 part yarrow leaves

Add 1 cup (250 ml) of boiling water to 1 tablespoon (15 g) of herbal mixture. Cover and steep for 15 minutes. Strain. Take ¹/₂ cup (125 ml) 3 times daily, one-half hour before meals.

CARDIAC ARRHYTHMIA RECIPE 2

1 part lily of the valley leaves
1 part motherwort

Prepare and take as above. (Lily of the valley preparations should only be taken under the supervision of a qualified health-care professional.)

CARDIAC ARRHYTHMIA RECIPE 3

1 part lily of the valley leaves   1 part raspberries (dried)
1 part pheasant's eye

Prepare and take as above.

Hypotonia

Hypotonia affects nearly half of all adults more than fifty years of age to varying degrees. In hypotonia, the muscular tension of the arteries relaxes, which can impair the flow of blood into the heart. A number of factors can cause hypotonia, including genetic predisposition, chronic emotional stress and other psychoemotional disorders, insomnia, disturbances in local and regional blood circulation, and poor circulation in the brain. Vomiting, dizziness, and headache may accompany hypotonia.

In Russia, medical doctors choose from three different approaches in treating symptoms of hypotonia: herbal therapy used alone; therapy beginning with allopathic drugs, which are gradually replaced by herbal formulas; and a combination of allopathic medications and herbal remedies prescribed at the same time. Unlike other forms of cardiovascular disease, hypotonia may require at least five to six months of herbal therapy. If the results are achieved within three months, herbalists nonetheless recommend continuing the herbal treatment, although the doses can be reduced. If positive results are not achieved during the first several months, herbalists report that the dose can be doubled without causing adverse side effects. One of the main advantages of herbal formulas in the treatment of hypotonia is that they do not cause an immediate drop of blood pressure like some synthetic drugs, which can result in light headedness when getting out of bed in the morning or while standing in a fast-moving elevator.

As with other forms of cardiovascular disease, herbs with diuretic properties often make up a major part of the complex herbal recipes. Following are the most common herbal remedies for treating hypotonia.

HYPOTONIA RECIPE 1

1 part cudweed	1 part periwinkle
2 parts horsetail	1 part yarrow leaves

Add 1 cup (250 ml) of boiling water to 1 tablespoon (15 g) of herbal mixture. Steep for 10 minutes and strain. Take $^1/_4$ cup (60 ml) 3 times daily after meals.

HYPOTONIA RECIPE 2

1 part motherwort	1 part valerian roots
1 part cudweed	1 part peppermint
1 part skullcap	

Prepare as above. Take $^1/_3$ cup (80 ml) 3 times daily before meals.

HYPOTONIA RECIPE 3

3 parts cudweed	1 part birch leaves
2 parts hawthorn berries	1 part licorice roots
2 parts everlasting flowers	

Prepare as above. Take $^2/_3$ cup (240 ml) 3 times daily one-half hour before meals.

HYPOTONIA RECIPE 4

1 part carrot seeds	1 part valerian roots
1 part fennel seeds	1 part hawthorn berries
1 part cornflower	

Prepare as above. Take $^1/_4$ cup (60 ml) 4 times daily one-half hour before meals.

HYPOTONIA RECIPE 5

1 part garlic cloves (mashed)   1 part valerian roots
1 part hawthorn flowers   1 part horsetail
1 part hawthorn berries

Prepare as above. Take 1 cup (250 ml) 2 to 3 times daily before meals.

HYPOTONIA RECIPE 6

1 part periwinkle leaves   1 part valerian roots
3 parts skullcap   1 part thyme
3 parts hawthorn berries

Prepare as above but cover and allow to stand for 2 hours. Filter. Take ¹/₂ cup (125 ml) 3 times daily before meals.

Varicose Veins

Varicose veins, a common health problem primarily affecting the legs, are enlarged, twisted veins that often cause pain in the feet and ankles, as well as swelling and skin ulcers. If a vein is injured, severe bleeding can result. In acute cases, varicose veins be may surgically removed.

Herb therapy for varicose veins is not as successful as it is in treating other circulatory disorders. Nevertheless, Russian folk healers have developed a number of complex herbal formulas that help reduce the symptoms. They work best at specific stages of the problem: when symptoms first appear and after surgical treatment.

VARICOSE VEINS RECIPE

2 parts horse chestnut bark   3 parts milfoil
5 parts willow bark   3 parts rue leaves

Add 1 tablespoon (15 g) of herbal mix to 1 cup (250 ml) of boiling water. Boil gently (preferably in a water banya) for 30 minutes. Filter. Drink 1 cup 3 times daily for 1 month. This course of treatment can be extended for another month if needed.

Russian herbalists suggest that this recipe works best when used in conjunction with other forms of medical care, including allopathic medications, exercise, and other lifestyle changes as recommended by the physician.

Thrombophlebitis

If left untreated, varicose veins can develop into thrombophlebitis, the painful inflammation of a vein that can lead to the formation of a blood clot. To treat this potentially life-threatening problem, herbalists recommend using botanicals with anticoagulant properties, such as milfoil and everlasting. Like other problems involving the circulatory system, thrombophlebitis requires the attention of a physician.

THROMBOPHLEBITIS RECIPE 1

1 part yarrow leaves
4 parts everlasting leaves
   and flowers

2 parts birch leaves
2 parts chamomile flowers

Prepare as in the Varicose Veins Recipe above, but boil for only 5 minutes in the water banya. Allow to stand for 4 hours. Filter. Take ¹/₂ cup (125 ml) 3 times a day before meals.

THROMBOPHLEBITIS RECIPE 2

1 part horse chestnut bark
1 part chamomile flowers

1 part horsetail

Add 1 cup (250 ml) of boiling water to 2 tablespoons (30 g) of herbal mixture. Steep for 2 hours and strain. Take ¹/₃ cup (80 ml) 3 times a day before meals.

THROMBOPHLEBITIS RECIPE 3

1 part sage leaves
1 part chamomile flowers
1 part althaea roots

1 part flaxseeds
1 part calendula flowers

Mash 3 tablespoons of herbal mixture in ¹/₃ cup (80 ml) of boiling water. Steep for 30 minutes. Make a warm compress and place on inflamed area.

THROMBOPHLEBITIS RECIPE 4

3 parts horsetail
3 parts chamomile flowers

1 part St. Johnswort

Prepare as in Thrombophlebitis Recipe 1. Take ¹/₄ cup (60 ml) 3 times a day. Use the leftover liquid in a warm compress.

Hemorrhoids

Hemorrhoids are defined medically as "a mass of dilated tortuous veins" in the anus that are often itchy and painful. In addition to keeping the area clean, physicians often recommend hemorrhoid creams and stool softeners. In acute or chronic cases, surgical removal may be necessary.

Herbalists suggest that herbal treatment for hemorrhoids should not be limited to the recipes described in this section. Because a hemorrhoid can be classified as a type of varicose vein, herbalists suggest using some of the varicose vein or thrombophlebitis recipes as well. For instance, a patient can use Hemorrhoid Bath Recipe 3 plus Thrombophlebitis Recipe 3 once a day. In addition, the patient can adopt dietary measures that can help soften stools and promote regularity. These often include (but are not limited to) taking a teaspoonful (5 ml) of olive oil before bedtime and eating laxative fruits like fresh apples, fresh pears, and cooked prunes.

Many Russian physicians who use herbs in their practice have testified to the ability of complex herbal formulas to relieve hemorrhoids, especially when used at the onset of symptoms. However, they stress that hemorrhoidal symptoms can rarely be resolved with one course of treatment. Generally speaking, Russian herbalists recommend using these hemorrhoid recipes daily for 10 to 14 days. They also suggest that the patient try different recipes for each separate course of treatment (if necessary) rather than use just one over and over again.

Most of the herbs that help relieve hemorrhoids contain aperient, antiphlogistic, and coagulant properties. Herbalists suggest that the following complex remedies be taken internally as soon as symptoms appear.

HEMORRHOID RECIPE 1

1 part aniseed	2 parts licorice roots
1 part fennel seeds	1 part buckthorn leaves

Add 1 cup (250 ml) of boiling water to 1 tablespoon (15 g) of herbal mix. Steep for 10 minutes and strain. Take ⅓ cup (80 ml) after breakfast and another after dinner.

HEMORRHOID RECIPE 2

3 parts restharrow roots	1 part thyme seeds
1 part buckbean leaves	2 parts lemon balm leaves

Add 1 tablespoon (30 g) of herb to 1 cup (250 ml) of water. Heat in a water banya for 15 minutes. Steep until the mixture cools to room temperature. Filter. Take 1 cup (250 ml) after breakfast and another after dinner.

HEMORRHOID RECIPE 3

1 part dandelion	1 part yarrow leaves
2 parts calendula flowers	1 part buckbean leaves

Prepare and take as in Hemorrhoid Recipe 1.

HEMORRHOID RECIPE 4

4 parts restharrow roots	3 parts elecampane
2 parts sage	1 part nettle leaves
2 parts shepherd's purse	

Prepare as in Hemorrhoid Recipe 1. Take ¹/₂ cup (125 ml) 3 times daily after meals.

HEMORRHOID RECIPE 5

3 parts oak bark	4 parts chamomile flowers
3 parts flaxseeds	

Prepare and take as in Hemorrhoid Recipe 4.

In Russia, a number of commercially prepared hemorrhoidal ointments are available that use horse chestnut as the major therapeutic ingredient. If this is not available, herbalists recommend an herbal sitting bath, in which the patient sits in a basin containing a warm herbal infusion. Two to three quarts (2 to 3 liters) of the infusion are poured into the basin after it has been rinsed with warm water to heat it up. Generally speaking, the bath should be as hot as the patient can tolerate and be taken for 15 to 20 minutes at a time. Some herbalists recommend reserving an extra quart or liter of the infusion in a thermos bottle and adding it as the bath cools. After the bath, cover the exposed areas of the body (such as the back and legs) with

a comfortable bath towel or sheet. The following bath recipes are traditionally used to treat hemorrhoids, and can also be used to make a warm
compress.

HEMORRHOID BATH RECIPE 1

5 parts oak bark	2 parts restharrow roots
3 parts horsetail	

Add 15 tablespoons (225 g) of herbal mixture to 2 quarts (2
liters) of boiling water. Heat in a water banya for 30 minutes.
Strain. An additional quart (liter) of boiling water can be added
to the mixture once it is ready.

HEMORRHOID BATH RECIPE 2

1 part horse chestnut fruit	5 parts oak bark
3 parts chamomile flowers	2 parts plantain leaves

Add 4 tablespoons (60 g) of herbal mixture to 2 quarts (2 liters)
of boiling water. Prepare as above. Add an additional quart
(liter) of boiling water if desired.

HEMORRHOID BATH RECIPE 3

1 part yarrow leaves	1 part plantain leaves
1 part nettle leaves	1 part chamomile flowers
1 part oak bark	

Add 2 quarts (2 liters) of boiling water to 3 tablespoons (45 g) of
mixture. Prepare as above.

THE RESPIRATORY SYSTEM

❧❦❧

Russian herbal medicine classifies herbs used for the treatment of diseases of the respiratory passages according to their therapeutic actions: They include anti-inflammatories (birch, oak, St. Johnswort, coltsfoot, elecampane, raspberry, chamomile, elder), antispasmodics (carrot, plantain, chamomile, wild marjoram, thyme, licorice, linden), antiseptics (calendula, chamomile, plantain, elecampane, pine, sage, St. Johnswort, birch, juniper), antiallergics (birch, licorice, pansy), nutritionals (raspberry, bilberry, nettle, rowan), and expectorants (althaea, elecampane, coltsfoot, plantain, licorice, thyme).

Colds, Flu, and Related Infections

Colds and flu usually affect the mucous layers of the throat, bronchia, and windpipe. They can sometimes lead to a number of chronic diseases, including bronchitis, tonsillitis, and sinusitis. On rare occasions, they can even be followed by more serious lung infections like pneumonia.

Many of us experience several colds a year, and we know the symptoms well: chest or throat discomfort, runny nose, headache, and fever are among the most common. Some cold sufferers need to stay home and rest for at least one to two days, and choose from a wide variety of over-the-counter cold medicines to alleviate unpleasant cold symptoms. Cold sufferers are also told to drink at least eight glasses of liquids a day and consume fruits and vegetables that are high in vitamin C, such as oranges, grapefruit, and broccoli. Vitamin C supplements are also recommended.

Flu is far more intense than the common cold and the onset of symptoms occurs more rapidly. Chilliness, malaise, and severe head and body pain are common, along with cough and fever. After four or five days the patient gets better, unless pulmonary complications are present as well. Pain relievers, bed rest, and plenty of liquids are often suggested while the disease persists.

Over the centuries, Russian herbalists have developed a number of herbal recipes that can not only treat cold and flu symptoms, but can help prevent a cold or flu before the symptoms manifest fully. As my own childhood experience showed, using these recipes the evening of the onset of symptoms can relieve symptoms by the following morning. However, my grandmother told us to continue with the recipe for another day or two, just to be on the safe side. Remember that recovery time varies with each individual and the severity of symptoms.

COLD AND FLU RECIPE 1

1 part raspberry leaves   2 parts wild marjoram leaves
2 parts coltsfoot leaves

Add 1 cup (250 ml) of boiling water to 1 tablespoon (15 g) of herbal mixture. Steep for 10 minutes and strain. Take 1 cup (250 ml) after dinner and 1 before bedtime.

COLD AND FLU RECIPE 2

1 part raspberries   1 part aniseed
2 parts linden flowers   1 part coltsfoot leaves

Prepare as above. Take 1 cup (250 ml) 3 times a day between meals.

COLD AND FLU RECIPE 3

3 parts linden flowers
1 part licorice roots

Prepare as above. Take 1 cup (250 ml) 3 to 4 times a day between meals.

COLD AND FLU RECIPE 4

1 part linden flowers   1 part elder flowers
1 part peppermint leaves

Prepare as above. Take 1 cup (250 ml) 3 to 4 times daily between meals.

Cold and Flu Recipe 5

1 part linden flowers   1 part St. Johnswort
1 part plantain leaves

Add 1 cup (250 ml) of boiling water to 1½ teaspoons (7 g) of herbal mixture. Cover and steep for 4 hours. Strain. Take ½ cup (125 ml) 3 times daily before meals.

Cold and Flu Recipe 6

1 part thyme   1 part marjoram
2 parts chamomile flowers

Prepare and take as above.

Cold and Flu Recipe 7

1 part marjoram   2 parts coltsfoot
2 parts raspberries

Add 1 cup (250 ml) of boiling water to 1 teaspoon (5 g) of herbal mixture. Steep for about 15 minutes and strain. Drink 1 cup (250 ml) 4 times a day 30 minutes before meals.

Bronchitis

We will examine two types of bronchitis in this section. Both involve inflammation of the mucous membrane of the bronchi, the two main air passages leading from the trachea (throat) to the lungs.

Acute Bronchitis

Acute bronchitis is perhaps the most common form of bronchitis. Caused by a virus, infection often follows a bout with the common cold. Early symptoms include chilliness and general feelings of malaise, with soreness and feelings of constriction behind the sternum. The cough is at first dry and painful, and the patient later coughs up phlegm. There is often a slight fever present, which can reach up to 102°F (39.8°C).

Most physicians prescribe bed rest, steam inhalations, and antibiotics for bronchitis, although the following complex recipes have been found to help alleviate bronchitis symptoms when used either alone or in addition to allopathic medications like antibiotics and analgesics.

ACUTE BRONCHITIS RECIPE 1

> 5 parts pine buds   1 part plantain leaves
> 1 part licorice roots

> Pour 1 cup (250 ml) of boiling water into a thermos containing 1 tablespoon (15 g) of herbal mixture. Close and allow to stand for 10 hours. Strain. Take ¹/₄ cup (60 ml) 3 times daily.

ACUTE BRONCHITIS RECIPE 2

> 2 parts althaea roots   2 parts coltsfoot leaves
> 2 parts licorice roots   1 part fennel seeds

> Add 1 cup (250 ml) of boiling water to 1 teaspoon (5 g) of herbal mixture. Cover and steep for 3 hours. Strain. Take warm ¹/₄ cup (60 ml) 3 times a day, one-half hour before meals.

Chronic Bronchitis

Chronic bronchitis is characterized by secretions of mucus by the tracheo-bronchial tract. People suffering from this disorder cough for up to two months. Because a tumor or tuberculosis can cause similar symptoms, it is important to have a physician who specializes in pulmonary diseases diagnose the problem. There are a number of factors that can contribute to this disease, including smoking and climate—rainy, humid weather during the spring or fall often exacerbates chronic bronchitis. If an infection is present, a course of antibiotics is often prescribed by the physician. In addition to lots of rest, natural healers often recommend diets rich in fresh fruits and vegetables, including natural juices.

The following herbal formulas are used to treat chronic bronchitis in Russia. If chronic bronchitis is a recurring problem, herbalists recommend using the following remedies as a preventive approach as well during the spring or fall, the primary seasons that favor chronic bronchitis.

CHRONIC BRONCHITIS RECIPE 1

> 1 part coltsfoot leaves   4 parts primrose flowers
> 2 parts plantain leaves   3 parts horsetail

> Pour 1 cup (250 ml) of water at room temperature into a pot with 1¹/₂ teaspoons (7 g) of herbal mixture. Steep for 2 hours. Heat to a slow boil, and continue boiling for 5 minutes. Strain. Take ¹/₄ cup (60 ml) 5 to 6 times a day.

CHRONIC BRONCHITIS RECIPE 2

4 parts althaea roots   1 part fennel seeds
4 parts licorice roots   1 part linden flowers
2 parts coltsfoot leaves

Prepare and take as above.

CHRONIC BRONCHITIS RECIPE 3

2 parts coltsfoot leaves   1 part marjoram
2 parts chamomile flowers   2 parts elecampane leaves

Prepare as above. Take 1 cup (250 ml) 3 times a day after meals.

CHRONIC BRONCHITIS RECIPE 4

2 parts elecampane roots   3 parts thyme
2 parts calendula flowers   3 parts coltsfoot leaves
3 parts plantain

Add 1 cup (250 ml) of boiling water to 1 tablespoon (15 g) of herbal mixture. Steep for 1 hour and filter. Take 1 cup (250 ml) 3 times a day 30 minutes before mealtimes.

Bronchial Asthma

Asthma is a disease that obstructs the airways. Symptoms include breathing difficulties, tightness in the chest, wheezing, and coughing. During an asthma attack, the muscles of the airways that connect the mouth and throat to the lungs tighten up. Bronchial asthma is a common form of asthma caused by an allergic reaction to pollen, molds, dust, foods, or chemicals in the workplace.

Bronchial asthma is a serious yet reversible condition that requires the care of a qualified health professional, usually a physician who specializes in lung diseases or allergies. A major aspect of treatment involves identifying the allergin and taking steps to avoid it or removing it from the patient's diet or living and working environment. In addition to medications such as antihistamines and bronchodilators, Russian doctors often prescribe herbs as well. The following recipes are among those used by both official and folk herbalists in Russia.

BRONCHIAL ASTHMA RECIPE 1

1 part thyme
1 part valerian roots
1 part fennel seeds

1 part peppermint
1 part chamomile flowers

Add 1 cup (250 ml) of boiling water to 1 tablespoon (15 g) of herbal mixture. Steep for 10 minutes and strain. Take ½ cup (125 ml) twice a day plus 1 cup (250 ml) before bedtime.

BRONCHIAL ASTHMA RECIPE 2

1 part pine buds
1 part aniseed

1 part licorice roots
1 part dill seeds

Prepare as above but steep for 1 hour. Take warm ¼ cup (60 ml) 4 times daily.

BRONCHIAL ASTHMA RECIPE 3

1 part licorice roots
1 part pansy

3 parts thyme

Prepare as in Bronchial Asthma Recipe 1. Take ¼ cup (60 ml) 4 times a day.

Pneumonia

Pneumonia is a very serious disease that involves inflammation of the lungs caused by bacteria, viruses, or chemical irritants. Chest pain, high fever, chills, coughing, and bloody sputum are among the more common symptoms. Pneumonia is a life-threatening disease, and aggressive medical treatment is often necessary. Penicillin is the traditional drug of choice to combat pneumonia, although other antibiotics are often used. While this approach may well save the patient's life, powerful antibiotics can also compromise the immune system, leaving us open to a host of other health problems.

Although Russian physicians use aggressive treatments such as antibiotics like their Western counterparts, they also stress the importance of enhancing the patient's immune system through exercise, diet, and healing herbs.

PNEUMONIA RECIPE 1

2 parts althaea roots   1 part fennel seeds
2 parts licorice roots

Add 1 cup (250 ml) of boiling water to 1 teaspoon (5 g) of herbal mixture. Cover and steep for 3 hours. Strain. Take warm ¹/₃ cup (80 ml) every 3 hours.

PNEUMONIA RECIPE 2

4 parts coltsfoot leaves   3 parts licorice roots
3 parts plantain leaves   1 part linden flowers

Prepare and take as above.

PNEUMONIA RECIPE 3

1 part thyme   4 parts coltsfoot flowers
1 part fennel seeds   2 parts plantain leaves
1 part peppermint   2 parts licorice roots

Add 1 cup (250 ml) of boiling water to 1 tablespoon (15 g) of herbal mixture. Steep for 1 hour and strain. Take 1 cup (250 ml) 3 times daily 30 minutes before mealtimes.

THE FEMALE
REPRODUCTIVE SYSTEM

The female reproductive system is a miracle of creation. Made up in part by the ovaries (where both the hormone estrogen and the female sex cells or ova are created), and the uterus (the organ which stretches to accommodate a fetus), the female reproductive system receives sperm, protects and nurtures the developing fetus, and finally gives birth to the new baby. This miraculous system responds to cycles. The monthly menstrual cycle involves communication among the brain, ovaries, and uterus by way of hormones, a type of chemical messenger. While it ceases during pregnancy, it is a cyclic cleansing process that continues from the beginning of puberty until a woman reaches menopause. On the following pages, we will examine some potential irregularities of the female reproductive system and discuss how complex herbal formulas can help in normalizing them.

Menorrhagia

Menorrhagia is excessive uterine bleeding at the time of a woman's menstrual period. The bleeding can be excessive on a particular day or may go beyond the normal period of menstruation. It may be caused by a wide variety of factors, including systemic diseases like diabetes or hypertension. Menorrhagia can also be due to fibroid growths or pelvic inflammation. After a competent medical diagnosis, Russian herbalists recommend the following recipes to help treat this problem.

MENORRHAGIA RECIPE 1

1 part tormentil   1 part valerian roots
1 part yarrow

Add 1 tablespoon (15 g) of herbal mixture to a pot containing 1 cup (250 ml) of boiling water. Turn off heat, cover, and steep for 2 hours. Reheat to boiling, then reduce heat and simmer for a few seconds. Pour into a thermos bottle, close, and steep for 4 hours. Strain. Take 1 cup (250 ml) twice a day before meals.

MENORRHAGIA RECIPE 2

1 part oak bark   1 part tormentil roots
1 part plantain leaves   1 part yarrow
1 part raspberry leaves

Prepare as above. Take ¼ cup (60 ml) 4 times daily.

MENORRHAGIA RECIPE 3

2 parts yarrow   3 parts tormentil roots
2 parts shepherd's purse 2 parts oak bark

Prepare as above. Take 1 cup (250 ml) twice a day.

MENORRHAGIA RECIPE 4

4 parts yarrow leaves   3 parts shepherd's purse
4 parts tormentil roots   2 parts oak bark

Prepare as above. Take 1 cup (250 ml) in the morning and 1 in the evening.

MENORRHAGIA RECIPE 5

2 parts valerian roots   1 part tormentil roots
2 parts yarrow leaves

Prepare as above. Take ½ cup (125 ml) 4 times daily.

Menstrual Pain

The following recipes are recommended to help relieve pain, cramps, and spasms during normal menstruation.

MENSTRUAL PAIN RECIPE 1

2 parts chamomile flowers   1 part lily of the valley herb
2 parts lemon balm   1 part red clover flowers

Place 1 tablespoon (15 g) of mixture into a container and add 1 cup (250 ml) of boiling water. Cover, steep for 15 minutes, and filter. Take 1 cup twice a day. A course of treatment should begin 2 to 3 days before menstruation and end when the period is over.

MENSTRUAL PAIN RECIPE 2

2 parts chamomile flowers   1 part calendula flowers
1 part valerian roots   2 parts red clover flowers

Prepare and use as above.

Menopause

Menopause is sometimes accompanied by a variety of symptoms such as irritation, mood swings, insomnia, and dizziness. Some women experience pains in the chest, which doctors believe may be caused by heart disease.

In Russia, herbalists and other natural healers prescribe hydrotherapy and exercise for their ability to bring about increased relaxation. In addition, herb therapy is often recommended, but healers stress that the types of herbs to use depend on the symptoms. For example, a woman experiencing sudden increases in blood pressure that may be related to menopause might want to use complex herbal formulas that treat hypertonia in addition to those for menopause listed on the following pages.

MENOPAUSE RECIPE 1

1 part peppermint leaves   2 parts fennel seeds
1 part restharrow   3 parts linden flowers
1 part mugwort

Add 2 tablespoons (30 g) of herbal mixture to 2 cups (500 ml) of cold water. Cover and allow to stand for 2 hours. Heat to boiling, then reduce heat and simmer for a few seconds. Pour into a thermos, close, and steep for 2 hours. Strain. Take 1 cup (250 ml) in the morning and 1 in the evening before meals.

MENOPAUSE RECIPE 2

1 part restharrow   1 part valerian roots
1 part birch leaves   1 part peppermint leaves
1 part yarrow

Prepare and take as above.

MENOPAUSE RECIPE 3

1 part chamomile flowers   1 part peppermint leaves
1 part yarrow   1 part calendula flowers
1 part lemon balm

Add 1 tablespoon (15 g) of herbal mixture to 1 cup (250 ml) of cold water. Cover and allow to stand for 2 hours. Heat to boiling, then reduce heat and simmer for a few seconds. Pour into a thermos, close, and steep for 2 hours. Strain. Take $1/4$ cup (60 ml) 4 times a day.

The Skin and Musculoskeletal System

⚜

The Skin

The skin is the external covering of the body. It not only protects us from injuries, germs, and other toxins in the environment, but it holds our bodies together. The skin also aids in elimination, regulates body temperature, and prevents dehydration. As the largest organ of the body, the skin is our major sense organ and is responsible for our getting enough vitamin D.

The skin is often a mirror of our health. When we see a person with pale, sallow, or blotchy skin, we often conclude that he or she is unhealthy; by contrast, clear, smooth, and radiant skin reflects good health and vitality.

Dermatitis, Eczema, and Neurodermatitis

Dermatitis, or skin inflammation, is the most common type of skin disease. In general, dermatitis symptoms include redness, itching, and skin lesions, which can be caused by poison ivy, chemicals, sunlight, or allergy.

Eczema is often more severe than "garden variety" dermatitis and is characterized by a variety of unpleasant symptoms, including pustules, skin lesions, itchy scabs, dry or watery discharge, and itching or burning. It is often difficult to heal.

Neurodermatitis is a type of skin inflammation partly due to emotional causes. It is characterized by itching and is often difficult to treat.

There are a number of allopathic treatments for these diseases, which should be treated by a qualified dermatologist or a medical specialist in skin diseases. A good diagnosis would be based on the patient's history, and an awareness of any other problems (be they medical, work-related, or psychological) that may be contributing to the skin condition.

Numerous allopathic pharmaceuticals have been developed over the years to treat these skin diseases, but many Russian physicians have seen good results with herbal therapy and often recommend it to their patients. Although skin diseases manifest on the body's surface, herbalists have developed a number of preparations that help the body to heal from the inside out. The following complex herbal recipes are designed to treat skin diseases like dermatitis, eczema, and neurodermatitis.

DERMATITIS/ECZEMA RECIPE 1

1 part yarrow
1 part peppermint leaves
1 part mugwort
2 parts licorice roots

2 parts marjoram
2 parts bilberry leaves
1 part buckbean leaves

Add 1 tablespoon (15 g) of herbal mixture to 1 cup (250 ml) of boiling water. Pour into a thermos, close, and steep for 2 hours. Strain. Take ¹/₄ cup (60 ml) 3 times daily.

DERMATITIS/ECZEMA RECIPE 2

1 part chamomile flowers
1 part peppermint leaves
1 part bilberry leaves

1 part licorice roots
3 parts valerian roots
1 part sweet flag roots

Prepare as above. Take ¹/₂ cup (125 ml) 3 times daily.

DERMATITIS/ECZEMA RECIPE 3

5 parts dandelion roots
3 parts fennel seeds
1 part calendula flowers
1 part thyme seeds

1 part kidney beans (cooked, mashed)
1 part buckbean leaves

Prepare as above. Take ¹/₂ cup (125 ml) 4 times daily.

DERMATITIS/ECZEMA RECIPE 4

1 part licorice roots
1 part sweet flag roots
3 parts marjoram herb

1 part mugwort leaves
1 part peppermint leaves
5 parts thyme seeds

Prepare as above. Take ¹/₂ cup (125 ml) 3 times daily 10 to 15 minutes before meals.

DERMATITIS/ECZEMA RECIPE 5

1 part marjoram
7 parts birch leaves
1 part coriander seeds

4 parts celandine
4 parts motherwort

Prepare as above. Take ¹/₄ cup (60 ml) 4 times a day before meals.

Lichen Planus

Lichen planus is an inflammatory skin disease of unknown origin that can take many forms. Symptoms may include the formation of tiny papules, rough scaly patches, redness, and itching. Russian doctors have often treated this problem with topical ointments with some degree of success. However, herbalists have developed a number of recipes to be taken internally that they have found successful in treating this skin disease.

LICHEN PLANUS RECIPE 1

2 parts elecampane
1 part celandine roots

1 part lemon balm
1 part peppermint leaves

Add 2 tablespoons (30 g) of herbal mixture to a pot containing 2 cups (500 ml) of water. Heat to boiling, then reduce heat and simmer gently for 5 minutes. Pour into a thermos, close, and steep for 2 hours. Filter. Take ¹/₂ cup (125 ml) 4 times a day.

LICHEN PLANUS RECIPE 2

1 part valerian roots
1 part plantain leaves
1 part mugwort

1 part motherwort
1 part peppermint leaves

Prepare as above. Take ¹/₃ cup (80 ml) 4 times a day.

LICHEN PLANUS RECIPE 3

> 1 part calendula flowers
> 1 part sage leaves

> Add 1 cup (250 ml) of boiling water to 1 teaspoon (5 g) of herbal mixture. Cover and steep for 15 minutes.
> Prepare 1 tablespoon (15 ml) of common plantain juice according to instructions found in the herb description (see page 115). Approximately 10 minutes after ingesting the juice, drink $^1/_4$ cup (60 ml) of the calendula and sage infusion. Prepare $^1/_4$ cup (60 ml) of the clinker polypore extract according to instructions found in the herb description (see page 56). Drink this extract 30 minutes after the calendula and sage infusion. This process should be repeated 3 times a day.

Psoriasis

Psoriasis is a common type of dermatitis characterized by itchy, dry, and scaly skin. It is generally treated with topical pharmaceutical preparations to reduce inflammation and to make the patient more comfortable. Many Russian dermatologists prefer herbal treatment for psoriasis and have developed a number of complex recipes in conjunction with clinker polypore extract. One standard prescription is to take $^1/_2$ cup (125 ml) of the clinker extract 3 times a day either 30 minutes before or 30 minutes after taking one of the following recipes.

PSORIASIS RECIPE 1

> 1 part primrose roots   1 part valerian roots
> 1 part buckbean leaves   2 parts dandelion flowers
>   and leaves

> Add 1 tablespoon (15 g) of herbal mixture to 1 cup (250 ml) of boiling water. Pour into a thermos, close, and steep for 2 hours. Strain. Take 1 cup (250 ml) 3 times daily.

PSORIASIS RECIPE 2

> 1 part licorice roots   1 part St. Johnswort
> 1 part dandelion flowers
>   and leaves

> Prepare as above. Take $^1/_4$ cup (60 ml) 3 times a day.

PSORIASIS RECIPE 3

1 part valerian roots   1 part peppermint leaves

2 parts licorice roots

Prepare as above. Take 1 cup (250 ml) at dinnertime and another $^1/_2$ cup (125 ml) before bedtime.

Herbal Baths

Using complex herbal recipes as a bath for treating skin diseases is one of the most complicated aspects of Russian herbal medicine. In my years of research reviewing the herbal literature and in interviewing dozens of patients and dermatologists, I was not able to identify one universal complex herbal recipe that was 100 percent effective in treating patients with skin diseases.

While new recipes are still being created in Russia today, a number of the already-popular ones are included here. Although some recipes will work well for certain people, others may not be as helpful. However, they are all safe and should cause no adverse side effects.

The standard form of preparing the following herbal bath recipes is to add 1 cup (250 ml) of the herbal mixture to 3 quarts (3 liters) of cold water. Cover and allow to stand for 2 hours. Then heat the water slowly to boiling and simmer for 5 minutes. Remove from heat, cover, and steep for another 2 to 4 hours. Strain out the larger particles while leaving the smaller ones in the mixture. Pour into a bathtub filled with water. Bathwater should be between 90 and 95°F (32 and 35°C).

Lie in the bath for 15 minutes. If you have a source of warm air in the bathroom, stand under or in front of it for 5 to 10 minutes and allow it to dry you. If not, gently pat your skin dry with a soft clean towel, or simply put on a clean cotton terry-cloth bathrobe.

Herbalists recommend taking this bath every evening just before bedtime. If condition improves within 2 to 3 weeks, reduce the bathing frequency to 5 times weekly for another 3 weeks, and then 2 to 3 times weekly after that.

ANTI-ITCHING AND SOOTHING BATH RECIPE 1

1 part horsetail   1 part oak bark

2 parts burdock roots   1 part lily of the valley

ANTI-ITCHING AND SOOTHING BATH RECIPE 2

2 parts lily of the valley   1 part plantain leaves
1 part chamomile flowers

ANTISEPTIC, ANTI-INFLAMMATION, AND ASTRINGENT BATH RECIPE 1

1 part St. Johnswort   1 part calendula flowers
3 parts celandine herb

ANTISEPTIC, ANTI-INFLAMMATION, AND ASTRINGENT BATH RECIPE 2

1 part sage   2 parts elecampane roots
1 part birch leaves   1 part celandine

ANTISEPTIC, ANTI-INFLAMMATION, AND ASTRINGENT BATH RECIPE 3

2 parts birch leaves   1 part St. Johnswort
1 part celandine

LICHEN PLANUS BATH RECIPE 1

1 part lemon balm   1 part peppermint leaves
1 part celandine

LICHEN PLANUS BATH RECIPE 2

1 part motherwort   1 part valerian roots
1 part lemon balm

PSORIASIS BATH RECIPE

1 part celandine leaves
1 part juniper berries

Russian herbalists suggest adding 6 cups (1¹/₂ liters) of clinker polypore extract to this bath to obtain better results.

Musculoskeletal System and Osteoarthritis

Osteoarthritis is one of the most common health problems that affects the musculoskeletal system. It causes chronic pain, swelling, and limited movement in joints throughout the body. It is often accompanied by deformities in the bone structure, usually in the fingers. Arthritis limits everyday activities such as walking, dressing, or bathing, which often leads to feelings of hopelessness and depression.

Although there are over one hundred different forms of arthritis, osteoarthritis is the most common of three prevalent types. The others are fibromyalgia and rheumatoid arthritis. Osteoarthritis is a degenerative joint disease in which the cartilage that covers the ends of bones in the joint deteriorates, causing pain and loss of movement as bone begins to rub against bone. In fibromyalgia, widespread pain affects the muscles and attachments to the bone. Rheumatoid arthritis is an autoimmune disease, in which the joint lining becomes inflamed as part of the body's immune system activity. The chronic inflammation causes deterioration of the joint as well as pain and limited movement. Scientists have not yet found a specific cause for most types of arthritis, and the actual disease process varies according to the form of arthritis the patient has.

Nearly forty million Americans have some form of arthritis, with the majority suffering from osteoarthritis. Three million suffer symptoms severe enough to be considered disabled. Although primarily affecting adults over the age of forty-five, arthritis can be found in people of all age groups, including children. Nearly two-thirds of arthritis sufferers are women.

There is no known cure for osteoarthritis. The primary goal of medical treatment is to manage the symptoms of pain, swelling, and joint stiffness. Most protocols include a combination of medication, exercise, rest, the use of heat and cold, joint protection techniques, and surgery on rare occasions.

Herbalists have been treating people suffering from osteoarthritis for centuries. While Russian herbalists do not claim to be able to cure this chronic disease, both single herbs (such as burdock, comfrey, and restharrow) and complex recipes have been found to relieve many of the painful symptoms that arthritis sufferers experience. The two complex recipes that follow are among the most successful in treating this common health problem.

OSTEOARTHRITIS RECIPE 1

1 part dandelion flowers and leaves	4 parts nettle leaves
1 part St. Johnswort	1 part birch leaves

Add 1 tablespoon (15 g) of herbal mixture to 2 cups (500 ml) of cold water. Cover and let stand for 2 hours. Heat to boiling, then reduce heat and simmer for 5 minutes. Pour into a thermos, close, and steep for 4 hours. Take $1/2$ cup (125 ml) 3 times daily before meals.

OSTEOARTHRITIS RECIPE 2

3 parts nettle leaves	1 part burdock roots
1 part pansy	

Prepare and take as above.

THE IMMUNE SYSTEM

The body's immune system is a marvel of intelligence, strength, and versatility. It is made up of millions of distinct organs, tissues, and cells that are distributed throughout the body and work together to protect us from external microorganisms, such as bacteria, viruses, and parasites.

In addition to the skin, which shields the body from invading microorganisms, our respiratory system helps keep out bacteria and germs through sneezing, coughing, or trapping irritants in nasal hairs. In addition, the mucous membranes of the respiratory and digestive tracts contain *macrophages*, which detect, envelop, and destroy bacteria and cellular debris, and *antibodies*, which specifically combine with bacteria and bacterial toxins (called *antigens*) and neutralize them.

The thymus gland—believed to be the major component of the immune system—produces T-lymphocytes, white blood cells that control cell-mediated immunity and help the body fight off disease. The spleen also produces lymphocytes and destroys old and deficient red blood cells. In addition, the body produces specific chemicals that enhance immunity, including interferon and interleukin. They help activate white blood cells and kill bacteria, viruses, and fungi. Generally speaking, the stronger our immune system, the better we can protect ourselves from infection and disease.

Over the past few years, scientists have focused on a number of factors that adversely influence immune response. Excessive alcohol or sugar consumption, tobacco use, exposure to chemical toxins (including cigarette smoke, pesticides in food, and other environmental pollutants), high blood cholesterol and triglyceride levels, and certain medications (such as antibiotics) can decrease immune function. Psychological factors include chronic stress and depression. Heredity also plays a role in our basic level of immune response.

While there is not much we can do about our heredity, there are many factors that enhance immune response. Regular exercise, adequate rest, deep rhythmic breathing, and a positive mental attitude can easily become a part of our daily routine. A well-balanced diet—including generous amounts of fresh fruits and vegetables, whole grains and cereals, and legumes (such as soy products)—is vital for supporting all body processes, including immune response. Virtually all vitamins and minerals contribute to proper immune function, especially vitamin A, vitamin B_6 (pyridoxine), vitamin C, vitamin E, and zinc. Vitamin B_6, for example, is found in more than sixty different enzymes found in the body, many of which are involved in immune function. Vitamin C is a major component of white blood cells, particularly lymphocytes.

In Russia, the use of herbs to strengthen the body's immune system was not studied until very recently. Traditional folk herbalists did not study the scientific basis of why certain herbs helped the body heal. They only saw the positive results.

Recent investigations in Russia have led physicians to classify herbs that work specifically with the immune system into three basic categories:

1. Body tonics. A number of herbs, such as hawthorn, nettle, and rose hips (very rich in vitamin C) have a tonic effect on the body and provide strength and support to the immune system as a whole.
2. Immune system stimulators and restorers. Although much research needs to be done, it is believed that other herbs, such as horsetail, chaga, and ginseng, help restore the immune system at a molecular level and stimulate specific immune reactions in cases of diseases like cancer and AIDS.
3. Antiallergics. Some herbs, like calendula and pansy, work well with allergies. As we will see later on, allergic reactions take place when the immune system overreacts to an otherwise harmless substance, like pollen. These herbs help the immune system deal more appropriately with these substances.

The following recipes provide general support for the immune system. They can be used to promote wellness or to help the body heal itself during periods of disease.

IMMUNE TONIC 1

1 part hawthorn	1 part plantain leaves
2 parts rose hips	1 part calendula flowers

Add 1 tablespoon (15 g) of herbal mixture to 1 cup (250 ml) of boiling water. Pour into a thermos, close, and steep for 2 hours. Strain. Take 1 cup (250 ml) 3 times daily.

IMMUNE TONIC 2

2 parts hawthorn	1 part nettle
1 part rose hips	1 part St. Johnswort root

Prepare and take as above.

IMMUNE TONIC 3

1 part chamomile flowers	1 part rose hips
1 part horsetail stems	

Prepare and take as above.

IMMUNE STIMULATOR/RESTORER RECIPE 1

2 parts horsetail stems (mashed)	1 part nettle leaves
1 part ginseng roots (mashed)	

The use of fresh herbs is best for this and the following recipes. Add 2 tablespoons (15 g) of mixture to 2 cups (500 ml) of cold water. Cover and let stand for 4 to 6 hours. Then heat to boiling and simmer gently for 10 mintues. Let stand for another hour and strain. Take ¹/₂ to 1 cup (125 to 250 ml) 2 to 3 times daily.

This and the following recipes may be used in combination with chaga. They can be used on alternate days or you can take chaga in the morning and one of these recipes at night.

IMMUNE STIMULATOR/RESTORER RECIPE 2

1 part horsetail stems (mashed)	1 part licorice roots
1 part nettle leaves	1 part rose hips

Prepare and use as above.

Immune Stimulator/Restorer Recipe 3

3 parts horsetail stems   1 part nettle leaves
   (mashed)   1 part birch leaves
1 part valerian roots

Prepare and take as above.

Allergies

An allergy is an overreaction of the immune system to a particular substance that causes no problems in nonallergic individuals. Because of a
genetic or other predisposing factor, the immune system of allergic individuals mistakenly identifies a harmless substance entering the body as a
threat to health. Substances that can trigger allergic reactions may include
pollen, dust, animal dander, smoke, fumes, and foods such as nuts, shell-
fish, and milk. Allergic reactions primarily affect the skin, the respiratory
system, and the blood vessels.

Physicians treat allergies by identifying the allergen (the substance that
produces an allergic reaction) and eliminating it from the patient's diet or
environment. In some cases, antihistamines are prescribed, which hinder
the body's response to allergens. For many Russians, herbal therapy is used
to treat allergies without the adverse side effects of antihistamines. Russian
herbalists recommend that those suffering from seasonal allergies try several different complex herbal recipes over the course of the year (or season)
to see which works best for their particular situation. As a preventive, the
best time to begin using these recipes is before the allergy season starts. You
can safely take any of these recipes during the entire allergy season if
needed.

Allergy Recipe 1

1 part licorice roots   2 parts plantain
1 part everlasting   1 part horsetail

Add 1¹/₂ teaspoons (7 g) of herbal mixture to 1 cup (250 ml) of
cold water. Cover and allow to stand for 2 hours. Bring to a boil,
then reduce heat and simmer gently for 5 minutes. Pour into a
thermos, close and steep for 4 hours. Take ¹/₄ cup (60 ml) 3 times
daily before meals.

ALLERGY RECIPE 2

1 part calendula flowers
1 part pansy

2 parts peppermint leaves
1 part elecampane roots

Prepare and take as above.

ALLERGY RECIPE 3

3 parts birch leaves
2 parts sage
1 part calendula flowers

1 part chamomile flowers
1 part pansy

Prepare and take as above.

ALLERGY RECIPE 4

1 part pansy
1 part chamomile flowers
2 parts valerian

2 parts marjoram
1 part horsetail

Prepare and take as above.

ALLERGY RECIPE 5

1 part pansy
1 part plantain

2 parts valerian roots
2 parts burdock roots

Prepare and take as above.

ALLERGY RECIPE 6

1 part licorice roots
1 part birch buds
1 part birch leaves

1 part valerian roots
1 part chamomile flowers
1 part peppermint leaves

Prepare and take as above.

MENTAL AND
EMOTIONAL HEALTH
❦

A wide variety of disorders are related to emotional stress, such as anxiety, fear, insomnia, and hysteria. Psychotherapy can help the individual understand and resolve the underlying causes of the problem (such as physical disease, financial worries, or difficulties in a relationship). However, herbal therapy may be able to help as well. Herbs contain chemicals that can relax the brain centers and help reduce the intensity of stressful episodes. Though not a cure in itself, herbal treatment can provide a calming "space" that enables the patient to initiate his or her own healing.

The list of psychological problems that respond to herbs is a long one. We will examine a number of common problems on the following pages that Russian healers often deal with and show which remedies seem to work best.

Insomnia

As many of us know firsthand, insomnia involves the inability to fall asleep or waking up during the night. It may result from psychological stress or the presence of other physical problems, including pain. There are many herbal treatments for insomnia, and Russian herbalists recommend the following complex recipes.

INSOMNIA RECIPE 1

1 part valerian roots   3 parts everlasting
3 parts motherwort

Add 1 tablespoon (15 g) of herbal mixture to a thermos containing 1 cup (250 ml) of boiling water. Close and steep for 12 hours.
Strain. Take ¼ cup (60 ml) 3 times a day, especially during
periods of anxiety or nervous tension.

INSOMNIA RECIPE 2

1 part dill seeds   1 part motherwort
1 part valerian roots   1 part thyme

Prepare as above. Take 1 cup (250 ml) as a warm tea before
bedtime.

Hysteria

Hysteria is a general psychological term pertaining to symptoms of emotional instability, alternate laughing and crying, a marked craving for sym-
pathy, and sensory disturbances. It often occurs during periods of extreme
emotional or physical stress.

In addition to having the patient lie down in a quiet room and applying
cold compresses to the head, physicians sometimes prescribe sedatives or
psychological treatment. Russian herbalists prescribe the following recipes
for this problem.

HYSTERIA RECIPE 1

1 part coriander seeds
2 parts motherwort

Add 1 cup (250 ml) of boiling water to 1 tablespoon (15 g) of
herbal mixture. Cover and let stand for 2 hours. Strain. Take 2
tablespoons (30 ml) 5 times a day.

HYSTERIA RECIPE 2

2 parts dandelion roots and leaves   1 part wild marjoram
1 part rue leaves

Prepare as above. Take ½ cup (125 ml) 3 times daily before
meals.

HYSTERIA RECIPE 3

1 part mugwort	1 part dandelion roots
1 part St. Johnswort	1 part valerian roots

Prepare as above. Take ¹/₄ cup (60 ml) 4 times a day.

Fear

Most of us know what fear is: an emotional reaction to an environmental threat, whether real or perceived. Much has been written about fear. People commonly fear pain, rejection, losing a job, and getting sick. A child may fear the dark or crossing the street. A soldier may experience fear before going into battle. In Russia, both physicians and herbalists consider fear to be an actual disease symptom and treat it with the following herbal formula.

FEAR RECIPE

3 parts mugwort	1 part valerian roots
3 parts everlasting	4 parts lemon balm

Add 1 tablespoon (15 g) of herbal mixture to a thermos containing 1 cup (250 ml) of boiling water. Steep for 2 hours and strain. Sip 2 tablespoons (30 ml) of this infusion every few hours during the course of the day. You can continue taking this remedy for up to 2 weeks.

Neurosis

Neurosis is another general term used to describe a psychological disorder involving anxiety, nervousness, hysteria, obsessive/compulsive thoughts and actions, fear, hypochondriasis, and reactive depression with no obvious physical cause. According to *Taber's Cyclopedic Medical Dictionary,* "In general a symptom due to a neurotic reaction to a situation is just as real to the patient as if it were due to organic disease."

Most of us have different neuroses at different times in our lives. Psychologists believe that they are due to unresolved internal conflicts that make it difficult for us to adjust easily to life's varied demands. If neurosis is a major problem in a person's life, psychotherapy is often recommended, either with or without sedatives or tranquilizers, which can have a variety of adverse side effects. Russian herbalists have found that the following herbal formulas can help those suffering from neurosis without the unwanted side effects of tranquilizers and other drugs.

NEUROSIS RECIPE 1

> 3 parts angelica roots
> 2 parts valerian roots
>
> Add 1 tablespoon (15 g) of herbal mixture to a thermos containing 1 cup (250 ml) of boiling water. Steep for 4 to 6 hours and strain. Sip 2 tablespoons (30 ml) of this infusion 4 times a day.

NEUROSIS RECIPE 2

> 1 part hawthorn berries   1 part valerian roots
> 1 part yarrow
>
> Prepare as above. Take 1 cup (250 ml) twice a day.

NEUROSIS RECIPE 3

> 1 part chamomile flowers   1 part lily of the valley flowers
> 1 part althaea roots
>
> Prepare as above. Take 2 tablespoons (30 ml) 4 times daily. This is often used as a calmative for children 6 years and older, with a recommended dosage of 1 tablespoon (15 g) twice a day. A course of treatment should not exceed 3 weeks.

NEUROSIS RECIPE 4

> 1 part lily of the valley   3 parts peppermint leaves
>   flowers   4 parts valerian roots
> 2 parts dill seeds
>
> Add 1 teaspoon (5 g) of herbal mixture to a thermos containing 1 cup (250 ml) of boiling water. Steep for 4 to 6 hours and strain. Take ¹/₂ cup (125 ml) 3 times a day.

NEUROSIS RECIPE 5

1 part chamomile flowers	1 part everlasting
3 parts motherwort	1 part hawthorn flowers

Add 1 tablespoon (15 ml) of herbal mixture into a thermos containing 1 cup (250 ml) of boiling water. Steep for 4 to 6 hours and strain. Take ¹/₂ cup (125 ml) 3 times a day. This recipe is recommended for persons whose neurosis is accompanied or followed by dizziness, shortness of breath, or both.

Desire Disorders

There are physical, energetic, and psychological causes to so-called desire disorders, which include low sexual desire, inhibited sexual excitement, and inhibition of arousal. Stress, communication problems, and unresolved difficulties in the relationship all play an important role in sexual desire. The following herbal preparations are used to stimulate sexual function when "the mind is willing but the flesh is weak."

SEXUAL FUNCTION RECIPE 1

1 part St. Johnswort herb
1 part sweet flag roots

Add 1¹/₂ teaspoons (7 g) of herbal mixture to 1 cup (250 ml) of cold water. Cover and let stand for 2 hours. Heat to boiling, then reduce heat and simmer for 5 minutes. Pour into a thermos, close, and steep for 4 hours. Take ¹/₄ cup (60 ml) 4 times daily.

SEXUAL FUNCTION RECIPE 2

2 parts motherwort	1 part dandelion roots
1 part calendula flowers	

Add two tablespoons (30 g) of herbal mixture to 2 cups (500 ml) of cold water. Cover and allow to stand for 2 hours. Heat to boiling, then reduce heat and simmer for a few seconds. Pour into a thermos, close, and steep for 2 hours. Strain. Take ¹/₂ cup (125 ml) 3 times a day.

GLOSSARY

❦

The following terms are used in this book to describe the medicinal action of herbs and their combinations.

Alterative: an agent that produces a gradual beneficial effect on the body and mind.

Analgesic: a medicine or herb that relieves pain.

Anesthetic: an agent that produces insensitivity to pain.

Anodyne: a medicine or herb that relieves pain.

Anthelmintic: an agent that kills or expels parasitic intestinal worms.

Antibacterial: a substance that destroys bacteria or stops its growth.

Antibiotic: a substance that inhibits the growth of or kills microorganisms.

Anticatarrhal: an agent that relieves catarrh, or severe spells of dry cough.

Anticoagulant: an agent that prevents or inhibits the coagulation of blood.

Antidiabetic: something that helps to prevent or alleviate symptoms of diabetes.

Antidiarrheal: something that prevents or alleviate symptoms of diarrhea.

Antiemetic: a substance that will prevent or relieve vomiting or nausea.

Antifungal: a substance that destroys or stops the formation of fungi such as yeasts.

Antihistamine: a drug used to treat symptoms caused by allergies such as hay fever.

Antihydrotic: a substance that prevents or decreases perspiration.

Antihypertensive: an agent that reduces high blood pressure.

Anti-inflammatory: a substance that reduces inflammation or its effects.

Anti-irritant: something that reduces irritation or abnormal sensitivity.

Antilithic: an agent that prevents the formation of or helps dissolve stones in the urinary or biliary tracts.

Antimicrobial: a substance that destroys or stops the development of germs and bacteria.

Antiparasitic: a substance that kills parasites.

Antiphlogistic: a substance that relieves inflammation.

Antipyretic: an agent that reduces fever.

Antisclerotic: an agent which prevents or treats hardening of the arteries.

Antiseptic: an agent that prevents the growth of germs and bacteria.

Antispasmodic: an agent that relieves spasms and cramps.

Antitussive: something that relieves or prevents coughing.

Aperient: a very mild laxative.

Appetizer: an agent that stimulates the appetite.

Aromatic: a substance that has an agreeable odor.

Astringent: an agent that contracts organic tissue, thus reducing hemorrhages or body secretions.

Calmative: an agent that acts as a mild sedative.

Cardiac: an agent that has a tonic or restorative effect on the heart.

Carminative: an agent that removes or expels gas from the intestines.

Cathartic: a strong purgative that empties the bowels.

Caustic: a substance that is corrosive and can destroy living tissue.

Cholagogue: an agent that stimulates the flow of bile into the intestines.

Coagulant: an agent that causes blood to clot.

Demulcent: an agent that soothes or softens irritated skin or mucous membranes.

Depurative: something that promotes body cleansing.

Diaphoretic: an agent that promotes perspiration.

Digestive: an agent that promotes digestion.

Disinfectant: an agent that cleans infection and prevents the growth of germs and bacteria.

Diuretic: an agent that increases the production and elimination of urine.

Emetic: an agent that produces vomiting.

Emmenagogue: an agent that promotes or assists menstrual flow.

Emollient: an agent that softens or soothes the skin when applied locally.

Expectorant: an agent that facilitates the removal of mucus from the respiratory passages.

Febrifuge: an agent that reduces fever.

Galactagogue: an agent that promotes the secretion of milk.

Germifuge: an agent that reduces or eliminates the presence of germs.

Hemostatic: an agent that stops bleeding.

Hepatic: a substance that benefits liver function.

Hydragogue: an agent that promotes the watery evacuation of the bowels.

Hypnotic: an agent that induces sleep or helps dull the senses.

Immune potentiator: an agent that enhances the functioning of the immune system or promotes immunity.

Laxative: an agent that loosens and promotes the evacuation of the bowels.

Mucilaginous: having a gelatinous or sticky consistency.

Nervine: an agent having a calming or soothing effect on the nerves.

Purgative: an agent that promotes rapid evacuation of the bowels.

Purifier: an agent that cleanses, such as cleansing the blood.

Refrigerant: an agent that cools the body or reduces fever.

Rubefacient: an agent that reddens the skin.

Sedative: an agent that exerts a soothing, calming, or tranquilizing effect.

Soporific: a substance that induces sleep.

Spasmodic: a substance that promotes spasm.

Stimulant: any agent that increases functional activity of the body's physiological processes.

Stomachic: an agent that stimulates or tones the stomach.

Styptic: an agent that stops bleeding or hemorrhage.

Sudorific: an agent that promotes perspiration.

Tonic: an agent that increases the body's strength and tone.

Vasoconstrictor: an agent that constricts the blood vessels.

Vasodilator: an agent that dilates the blood vessels.

Vermicide: an agent that kills intestinal worms.

Vermifuge: an agent that expels intestinal worms.

Virucidal: the ability of a substance to kill viruses.

Vulnerary: an agent used to assist the healing of wounds.

BIBLIOGRAPHY

Books in English

Altman, Nathaniel. *Sacred Trees*. San Francisco: Sierra Club Books, 1994.

Buchman, Dian Dincin. *Herbal Medicine*. London: The Herb Society / Rider, 1987.

Culpeper, Nicholas. *Culpeper's Complete Herbal*. London: W. Foulsham, n.d.

Grieve, M. *A Modern Herbal*. 1931. Reprint, New York: Dover Publications, 1972.

Hoffman, David. *The New Holistic Herbal*. Shaftsbury, England: Element Books, 1990.

Lust, John. *The Herb Book*. New York: Bantam Books, 1974.

Mills, Simon. *Out of the Earth*. London: Viking Arcana, 1991.

Sanecki, Kay N. *The Complete Book of Herbs*. New York: Macmillan, 1974.

Santillo, Humbart. *Natural Healing with Herbs*. Prescott Valley, Ariz.: Holm Press, 1985.

Vogel, H. C. A. *The Nature Doctor*. New Canaan, Conn.: Keats Publishing, 1991.

Books in Russian (titles are translated into English)

Bogoyavlenky, N. A. *Old Russian Doctoring in the Eleventh and Twelfth Centuries*. Moscow: Goscomisdat, 1960.

Gammerman, A. F., et al. *The Herbs*. Moscow: Visshaya Shkola, 1983.

Kazarinova, N. V., et al. *The Herbs of Siberia Used for Cardiovascular Diseases.* Novosebirsk: Sibirskoe Otdelenie, 1991.

Korchan, V. L., and K. B. Kulemsa. *Secrets of Folk Medicine.* Moscow: Kredo, 1992.

Korshikov, B. M., et al. *Collection of Herbs.* Minsk: Uradzhai, 1977.

Krilov, A. A., et al. *Phytotherapy Used in Complex Treatment of the Diseases of the Internal Organs.* Kiev: Zdorovie, 1992.

Ladinina, E. H., and R. S. Morozova. *Herbs in Modern Medicine.* Kondopoga: Goscomizdat of KASSR, 1990.

Mahluk, V. N. *The Herbs in Folk Medicine.* Saratov: Goscomizdat, 1967.

Nosal, M. A., and E. M. Nosal. *The Herbs and Directions for Use in Folk Medicine.* Kiev: Gosmedizdat, 1958.

Pashinsky, V. G. *Herbs Used for Stomach and Duodenal Ulcers.* Odessa: Variant, 1990.

Pastushenkov, L.V., et al. *The Use of Herbs in Folk Medicine and in Everyday Life.* St. Petersburg: Lenizdat, 1990.

Perevozchenko, E. E. *Herbs in Modern Medicine.* Kiev: Obchestvo Znani, 1990.

Severova, E. Y. *Non-Specific Reactions of Patients on Herbal Remedies.* Moscow: Medicina, 1969.

Shass, E. U. *Phytotherapy.* Moscow: Academy of Medical Science of the USSR, 1952.

Sinyakov, A. F. *Tops and Roots.* Moscow: Phys. Culture and Sport, 1992.

Smirnov, A. *The World of Herbs.* Moscow: Molodaya Guardia, 1988.

Tomilin, S. A. *Phytotherapy Used by the Village Doctors.* Kiev: Gosmedizdat, 1954.

Ushbaev, K. U., et al. *Health-Giving Herbs.* Alma-Ata: Goscomizdat of KSSR, 1976.

Vinogranov, V. M., et al. *Herbs Used for Cardiovascular Diseases.* St. Petersburg: Inanie, 1990.

Yagodka, V. S. *Herbs in Dermatology and Cosmetology.* Kiev: Naukova Dumka, 1992.

Zaharov, P. V., et al. *Official Matters in Herbs and Their Modes of Production* Tashkent: FAN, 1980.

Zhigar, M.P. *The World of Health-Giving Roots.* Minsk: Urazdai, 1991.

HERBAL SUPPLIERS

❦

United States

Aphrodisia
264 Bleecker Street
New York, NY 10014
(212) 989-6440
(212) 989-8027 (fax)

*Herbs in bulk, teas, oils, books. Send
list of needs.*

Artemis Herbs and Botanicals
175 Neilson Road
New Salem, MA 01364
(508) 544-7559
(508) 544-7486 (fax)

*Organic and wildcrafted herbs in
bulk, custom blended teas, oils.
Mail-order catalog.*

Companion Plants
7247 N. Coolville Ridge Road
Athens, OH 45701
(614) 592-4643
(614) 593-3092 (fax)
http://www.frognet.net/
companion_plants

*Herb seeds and plants. Wholesale
and retail. Mail-order catalog.*

Frontier Cooperative Herbs
P.O. Box 299
Norway, IA 52318
(800) 669-3275

*Herbs in bulk, extracts, custom for-
mulas. Mail-order catalog. Whole-
sale/retail.*

Genesis Farms
P.O. Box 42
Clearcreek, IN 47426
(812) 824-7524

*Herbs in bulk and as custom formu-
las. Mail-order catalog.*

Indiana Botanic Gardens, Inc.
P.O. Box 5
Hammond, IN 46325
Customer service: (800) 514-1068
Orders only: (800) 644-8327

*Herbs in bulk, capsules, teas. Mail-
order catalog.*

Liberty Seed Co.
461 Robinson Drive SE
P.O. Box 806
New Philadelphia, OH 44663
(330)364-1611
(330) 364-6415 (fax)

Seeds for herbs, vegetables, and flowers. Mail-order catalog.

Natural Herbal Extracts
432 Bolton Road
East Windsor, NJ 08520
(609) 448-8744

Herbal extracts, including herbal formulas. Mail-order catalog.

Nature's Way
10 Mountain Springs Parkway
P.O. Box 4000
Springville, Utah 84663
(800) 9-NATURE

Herbs in capsule form. Mail-order catalog.

Nichols Garden Nursery
1190 N. Pacific Highway
Albany, OR 97321
(541) 928-9280

Herb seeds, plants, bulk herbs, teas. Mail-order catalog.

Vitamin Discount Connection
35 North 8th Street
P.O. Box 1431
Indiana, PA 15701
(800) 848-2990

Herbs in bulk, extracts, capsules, and vitamins. Mail-order catalog.

The Vitamin Trader
6501 Fourth Street, NW
Albuquerque, NM 87107
(505) 344-6060; (800) 334-9310
(505) 345-7146 (fax)
http://www.vitamin-trader.com

Herbs in capsule form, tablets, and teas. Mail-order catalog. Name-brand vitamins at discount prices.

Wind River Herbs
P.O. Box 3876
Jackson, WY 83001
(800) 903-4372

Liquid extracts formulated by the noted British herbalist David Hoffmann.

Canada

L'Armoire aux Herbes, Inc.
375 Rang des Chutes
Ham Nord, Quebec G0P 1A0
(819) 344-2080

Herbs and correspondence courses.

Herboristerie Desjardins, Inc.
3303 St. Catherines Street E.
Montreal, Quebec H1W 2C5
(514) 522-4860

Herbs in bulk, teas.

Richters
357 Highway 47
Goodwood, Ontario L0C 1A0
(905) 640-6677
(905) 640-6641 (fax)
Herbs in bulk, plants, seeds, oils,
books. Mail-order catalog.

Australia

Erdman's Cottage Herbs
59 Maiden Street
Greenacre, NSW 2190
02-642-4008

Lillydale Herb Farm
61 Mangans Road
Lillyvale, Vic. 3140
03-735-0486

Meadows Herbs
Sims Road
Mt. Barker, SA 5251
08-388-1611

Melody Farm Nursery
616 Old Northern Road
Dural, NSW 2158
02-651-1176

Rose-World Nursery
Redland Bay Road
Victoria Point, Q. 4163
07-207-7350

Somerset Cottage
745 Old Northern Road
Dural, NSW 2158
02-84-2267

United Kingdom

Baldwins
171-173 Walworth Road
London SE17 1RW
0171-703-5550
0171-252-6264 (fax)
baldwins@dial.pipex.com
Herbs and oils.

Neal's Yard Natural Remedies
15 Neal's Yard
Covent Garden, London WC2H
9DP
0171-379-7222
0171-379-0705 (fax)
Natural cosmetics, herbs, essential
oils, homeopathic remedies, food
supplements.

Potters Herbal Supplies Ltd.
Leyland Mill Lane
Wigan, Lancashire WN1 2SB
10942-234761
10942-820255 (fax)
Herbal medicine manufacture.

Plant Index

Achillea millefolium, 149–150
Adonis vernalis, 115–116
Aesculus hippocastanum, 84–85
Alchemilla vulgaris, 94–95
alehoof. *See* ground ivy
Allium sativum, 78–80
althaea, 26–27
Althaea officinalis, 26–27
aloe, 24–25
Aloe vera, 24–25
amber. *See* St. Johnswort
anise, 29–30
anise plant. *See* anise
angelica, 28–29
Angelica archangelica, 28–29
Angelica atropurpurea, 28
Antheum graveolens, 68–69
Apocynaceae family, 114–115
arctium lappa, 44–45
Arctostaphylos uva-ursi, 143–144
arnica, 30–31
Arnica montana, 30–31
ass ear. *See* comfrey

balm mint. *See* lemon balm
barberry, 32–33
barley, 33–35
bean trefoil. *See* buckbean
bearberry. *See* uva ursi
bee balm. *See* lemon balm
Berberidaceae family, 32–33
Berberis vulgaris, 32–33
Betonica officinalis, 35–36
betony, 35–36
Betula alba, 38–39
Betulaceae family, 38–39
bilberry, 36–37, 44
birch canker polypore. *See* clinker polypore
bird's nest. *See* carrot (wild)
bistort, 40–41
bitterwort. *See* yellow gentian
black elder. *See* elder
blue balm. *See* lemon balm
blue pimpernel. *See* skullcap
bogbean. *See* buckbean
Boraginaceae family, 60–61
briar hip. *See* rose hips
briar rose. *See* rose hips
brideswort. *See* meadowsweet

broad-leafed plantain. *See* common plantain
buckbean, 41–42
buckeye. *See* horse chestnut
buckthorn, 42–43
bullsfoot. *See* coltsfoot
burdock, 44–45
burr seed. *See* burdock
butter rose. *See* cowslip

calendula, 46–47, 220
Calendula officinalis, 46–47
cammock. *See* restharrow
Caprifoliaceae family, 70–71
Capsella bursa-pastoris, 132–133
carrot (cultivated), 48–49
carrot (wild), 47–48
Caryophyllaceae family, 129–130
catsfoot. *See* ground ivy
celandine, 50–51
Cetraria islandica, 88–89
chaga, 220
Chamaenerion, 147–148
chamomile, 14, 51–53, 145
Chelidonium majus, 50–51
China rhubarb. *See* rhubarb
cinquefoil, 53–54
clinker polypore, 55–56
cockleburr. *See* burdock
coltsfoot, 59–60
comfrey, 60–61
common anise. *See* anise
common birch. *See* white birch
common chamomile. *See* chamomile
common plantain, 118–119
Compositae family, plants belonging to, 30–31, 44–45, 46–47, 51–53, 59–60, 66–68, 72–73, 73–74, 139–140, 149–150
Convallaria majalis, 98–99
coriander, 62–63
coriander seed. *See* coriander
Coriandrum sativum, 62–63
coughwort. *See* coltsfoot
cowslip, 63–64
Crataegeus oxyacantha, 83–84
Crataegeus sanguinea, 83
Cruciferae family, 132–133
cucumber, 65–66
Cucumis sativus, 65–66
Cucuribitaceae family, 65–66

cudweed. *See* everlasting
Cupressaceae family, 91–92
cure-all. *See* lemon balm

dandelion, 66–68
Daucus carota, 47–48, 48–49
dill, 68–69
Dioscorea caucasia, 146
Dioscoreaceae family, 146–147
Dioscorea deltoides, 146
Dioscorea nipponica, 146
Dioscorea villosa, 146–147
dog rose. *See* rose hips
dragonwort. *See* bistort
dropsy plant. *See* lemon balm

eastern white pine, 117
elder, 70–71
elecampane, 72–73
elfdock. *See* elecampane
English meadowsweet. *See* meadowsweet
English oak, 108–109
Epilobium angustifolium, 147–148
Equisetaceae family, 86–87
Equisetum arvense, 86–87
Ericaceae family, 143–144
eternal flower. *See* strawflower
European angelica. *See* angelica
European elder. *See* elder
European mountain ash. *See* rowan
everlasting, 14, 73–74

Fagaceae family, 108–109
false hellebore. *See* pheasant's eye
fennel, 75–76
Filipendula ulmaria, 103–105
fireweed. *See* willow herb
five-finger grass. *See* cinquefoil
five-leaf grass. *See* cinquefoil
flax, 77–78
Foeniculum vulgare, 75–76
fragrant valerian. *See* valerian

garden angelica. *See* angelica
garden balm. *See* lemon balm
garden sage. *See* sage
garden thyme. *See* thyme
garden violet. *See* pansy
garlic, 78–80
gentian. *See* yellow gentian
Gentianaceae family, 81–82
Gentiana lutea, 81–82
German chamomile. *See* chamomile
ginseng, 220
Glycyrrhiza glabra, 97–98
Gnaphalium uliginosu, 73–74

goatweed. *See* St. Johnswort
Graminaceae family, 33–35
greater celandine. *See* celandine
greater plantain. *See* common plantain
ground ivy, 89–90
gypsy weed. *See* speedwell

hawthorn, 83–84
haymaids. *See* ground ivy
healing herb. *See* comfrey
heart's ease. *See* pansy
Helichrysum arenarium, 139–140
helmet flower. *See* skullcap
Herniaria glabra, 129–130
hippocastanaceae, 84–85
hip tree. *See* rose hips
holigold. *See* calendula
hops, 145
Hordeum vulgare, 33–35
horse chestnut, 84–85, 198
horse elder. *See* elecampane
horsehoof. *See* coltsfoot
horsetail, 86–87, 220
horsetail grass. *See* horsetail
horsetail weed. *See* horsetail
huckleberry. *See* bilberry
Hungarian chamomile. *See* chamomile
Hypericaceae family, 137–138
Hypericum perforatum, 137–138

Iceland lichen. *See* Iceland moss
Iceland moss, 88–89
Inonotus obligus [Fr.] pil., 55–56
Inula helenium, 72–73

jaundice berry. *See* barberry
Johnny jump-up. *See* pansy
juniper, 91–92
Juniperus communis, 91–92
Juniperus oxycedrus, 92

kinnikinnick. *See* uva ursi
knitback. *See* comfrey
knitbone. *See* comfrey
knotweed, 92–93

Labiatae family, plants belonging to, 35–36,
    89–90, 102–103, 113–114, 130–131, 134–
    135, 140–141
lady's mantle, 94–95
Lamiaceae family, 95–96
large fennel. *See* fennel
Leguminosae family, plants belonging to, 97–
    98, 122–123
lemon balm, 95–96
licorice, 14, 97–98

licorice root. *See* licorice
life everlasting. *See* everlasting
Liliaceae family, plants belonging to, 24–25, 29–30, 78–80, 98–99
lily of the valley, 98–99
linaceae, 77–78
linden, 100–101
linseed. *See* flax
Linum usitatissimum, 77–78
low cudweed. *See* everlasting

mallards.*See* althaea
Malvacae family, 26–27
marigold. *See* calendula
marjoram, 102–103
marsh cudweed. *See* everlasting
marshmallow. *See* althaea
marsh marigold. *See* cowslip
marsh trefoil. *See* buckbean
mary bud. *See* calendula
Matricaria chamomilla, 51–53
may bush. *See* hawthorn
may tree. *See* hawthorn
meadowsweet, 103–105
melissa. *See* lemon balm
Melissa officinalis, 95–96
Mentha piperita, 113–114
Menyanthaceae family, 41–42
Menyanthes trifoliata, 41–42
milfoil. *See* yarrow
mortification root.*See* althaea
mountain tobacco. *See* arnica

nettle, 105–107
nosebleed. *See* yarrow

oak, 108–109
Onagracae family, 147–148
Ononis spinosa, 122–123
Origanum vulgare, 102–103
oxeye. *See* pheasant's eye

pale gentian. *See* yellow gentian
pansy, 110–111, 220
Papaveraceae family, 50–51
paper birch. *See* white birch
Papilonaceae family, 57–58
Parmeliaceae family, 88–89
parsley, 111–112
passionflower, 145
patience dock. *See* bistort
peppermint, 113–114
periwinkle, 114–115
Petroselinim crispum, 111–112
pheasant's eye, 115–116
pickpocket. *See* shepherd's purse

Pimpinella anisum, 29–30
Pinaceae family, 117–118
pine, 15, 117–118
Pinus strobus, 117–118
piperage. *See* barberry
plantaginaceae, 118–119
Plantago major, 118–119
Poloyporaceae family, 55–56
Polygonaceae family, plants belonging to, 40–41, 92–93, 123–124
Polygonum bistorta, 40–41
Polygonum bistortoides, 40
Polygonum hydropiper, 92–93
Poria obliqua, 55–56
Potentilla anserina, 53–54
Potentilla tormentilla, 142–143
primrose. *See* cowslip
Primulaceae family, 63–64
Primula veris, 63–64

Queen Anne's lace. *See* carrot (wild)
queen of the meadow. *See* meadowsweet
Quercus alba, 108–109
Quercus robur, 108–109
Quercus rubra, 108–109

ramsthorn. *See* buckthorn
Ranunculaceae family, 115–116
raspberry, 15, 120–121
red clover, 57–58
red legs. *See* bistort
red oak, 108–109
red sage. *See* sage
restharrow, 122–123
Rhamnaceae family, 42–43
Rhamnus cathartica, 42–43
Rheum palmatum, 123–124
rhubarb, 123–124
Rosa canina, 124–125
Rosaceae family, plants belonging to, 53–54, 83–84, 94–95, 103–105, 120–121, 124–125, 126–127, 142–143
rosebay willow herb. *See* willow herb
rose hips, 12, 124–125
rowan, 126–127
Rubus strigosus, 120–121
rue, 127–128
rupturewort, 129–130
Rutaceae family, 127–128
Ruta graveolens, 127–128

sage, 130–131
St. James's weed. *See* shepherd's purse
St. Johnswort, 13, 137–138
Salvia officinalis, 130–131
Sambucus canadensis, 71

Sambucus nigra, 70–71
Sambucus racemosa, 71
Scrophulariaceae family, 135–136
Scutellaria baicalensis, 134–135
shave grass. *See* horsetail
shepherd's knot. *See* tormentil
shepherd's purse, 132–133
silver birch. *See* white birch
skullcap, 134–135
smartweed. *See* knotweed
sorb apple. *See* rowan
Sorbus aucuparia, 126–127
sowberry. *See* barberry
Spanish chestnut. *See* horse chestnut
speedwell, 135–136
stepmother. *See* pansy
stinging nettle. *See* nettle
strawflower, 139–140
sweet balm. *See* lemon balm
sweet dock. *See* bistort
sweet fennel. *See* fennel
sweet licorice. *See* licorice
sweet vernal. *See* pheasant's eye
sweet wood. *See* licorice
Symphytum officinale, 60–61

Taraxacum officinale, 66–68
thousand weed. *See* yarrow
thyme, 13, 140–141
Thymus serpellum , 140–141
Thymus vulgaris, 140–141
Tiliaceae family, 100–101
Tilia cordata, 100–101
Tilia europea, 100–101
tormentil, 142–143
Tormentilla erecta, 142–143
Trifolium pratense, 57–58
Turkey rhubarb. *See* rhubarb
Tussilago farfara, 59–60

Umbelliferae family, plants belonging to, 28–
29, 47–48, 48–49, 62–63, 68–69, 75–76,
111–112
Urticaceae family, 105–107
Urtica dioica, 105–107
uva ursi, 143–144

Vacciniaceae family, 36–37
valerian, 144–145
valerianaceae, 144–145
Valeriana officinalis, 144–145
veronica. *See* speedwell
Veronica officinalis , 135–136
Vinca major, 114–115
Vinca minor, 114–115
Violaceae family, 110–111
Viola tricolor, 110–111

water pepper. *See* knotweed
waybread. *See* common plantain
white birch, 15, 38–39
white man's foot. *See* common plantain
white oak, 108–109
white pine, 117
whitethorn. *See* hawthorn
whortleberry. *See* bilberry
wild chamomile. *See* chamomile
wild clover. *See* red clover
wild fennel. *See* fennel
wild marjoram, 13
wild yam, 146–147
willow herb, 147–148
wolfsbane. *See* arnica

yarrow, 149–150
yellow gentian, 81–82

General Index

abdominal cramps, 75
abscesses, 31, 78, 103, 112
Academy of Sciences of the Soviet Union, 134
achellein, 149
Achilles, 149
acne, 106, 121
acute bronchitis, 29, 102, 202–203
acute cholecystitis, 49
acute gastritis, 52, 154–155
acute glomerulonephritis, 178–179
adrenal glands, 139
ague, 133
AIDS, 87, 220
Alanton, 72
albumens, 146
alcoholism, 141, 144
allergic dermatitis, 52, 110, 112
allergic dermatosis, 108
allergies, 222–223
alliinase, 79
allopathic medicine, 3, 5, 7, 149, 178, 202, 211–212
All-Union Institute of Herbs and Aromatherapy, 3, 11, 30, 46
Ambodisk-Maksimovich, V. M., 10
amenorrhea, 102
analgesic, 38, 43, 52, 62, 79, 140
anal irritation, 43
anemia, 48, 57, 63, 68, 87, 96, 107, 120, 142
anesthetic, 65, 96, 112, 127
anethole, 75
angelic water, 28
Anita's eyes, 135
anodyne, 26, 36, 44, 50, 52, 53, 62, 63, 74, 77, 89, 97, 113, 117, 120, 122, 137, 143
anthelmintic, 28, 34, 48, 65, 67, 72, 77, 104, 134
antiallergic, 220
antibacterial, 24, 28, 40, 46, 60, 72, 79, 88, 97, 104, 110, 113, 120
antibiotic, 79, 205
antibodies, 219
anticatarrhal, 74, 89
anticoagulant, 100, 146
antidiabetic, 89
antidiarrheal, 36, 60
antiemetic, 55, 88, 120
antifungal, 46
antigens, 219

antihistamine, 97
antihypertensive, 35, 134
anti-inflammatory, 40, 43, 50, 216
anti-irritant, 117
anti-itching remedies, 37, 215–216. *See also* itching
antilithic, 47
antimicrobial, 49, 140
antinomycosis, 141
antiparasitic, 79
antiphlogistic, 28, 32, 34, 41, 46, 52, 59, 60, 65, 72, 77, 86, 88, 89, 93, 97, 99, 102, 104, 106, 108, 112, 114, 117, 119, 120, 121, 134, 142, 143, 148, 149
antipyretic, 29, 31, 63, 67, 84, 120, 134
antisclerotic, 89, 120, 132, 146
antiseptic, 24, 32, 42, 44, 46, 62, 70, 74, 79, 91, 99, 112, 113, 137, 142, 143, 149, 216
antispasmodic, 29, 48, 50, 52, 53, 62, 69, 75, 95, 97, 102, 112, 113, 116, 119, 134, 137, 140, 145, 146, 148, 149
antitussive, 69
Anuta's eyes, 110
anxiety, 100, 113, 145
aperient, 44, 55, 65, 67, 70, 119, 121
apoplexy, 99
appetite, poor, 169–170. *See also* appetizer
appetizer, 27, 34, 35, 42, 48, 62, 67, 72. 81, 88, 89, 95, 96, 112, 113, 120, 128, 134, 135, 136, 149, 150
aromatherapy, 38
aromatic, 38, 75
arteriosclerosis, 70, 77, 79, 146, 185–187
arthritis, 39, 52, 70, 91, 104, 106, 110. *See also* joint disorders; osteoarthritis; rheumatism; rheumatoid arthritis
ascariasis, 34. *See also* intestinal worms
ascaris, 139. *See also* intestinal worms
Ashshiurbanipal of Assyria, King, 32
Asian-Arabic herbal system, 9
asses' herbs, 122
asthenia, 57
asthma, 35, 63, 70, 74, 96, 141, 143, 148
astringent, 32, 35, 36, 38, 40, 53, 59, 74, 84, 93, 104, 106, 108, 114, 120, 137, 140, 142, 143, 148, 149, 216
atherosclerosis, 36, 58, 67, 86, 102, 106, 110, 185
attention deficit disorder, 96
Averin, 110

bacillary dysentery, 104. *See also* dysentery
back pain, 28, 34, 39, 44, 70, 74
bacteria, 95
bad breath. *See* halitosis
balding. *See* hair: loss
banya. *See* water banya; Russian baths
banya's mold, 9
bark, 15–16
bear's berry, 143
bear's ear, 143
bedsores, 66, 108
bed-wetting, 141
befungin, 55
berries, 15
Bible, 65
bile: expelling, 50, 137; promoting flow of, 28, 31, 32, 38, 52, 65, 67, 84, 139, 150. *See also* gallbladder; liver
birthmarks, 66
bittering yellow, 81
blackheads, 66, 67, 110
bladder. *See* gallbladder; urinary bladder
bladder stones, 66, 143
bleeding, external, 54, 74. *See also* hemorrhage; menorrhagia; metrorrhagia
blood circulation, 32, 72, 93
blood coagulation, 32, 149
blood pressure, 32, 46, 72, 73, 74, 79, 83, 95, 114, 133, 134, 146, 150
blood sugar, 37, 79, 106, 112, 120
blood vessels, 84–85, 112, 133
body tonic, 39, 98, 220
boils, 52, 59, 24, 44, 88, 94, 96, 105. *See also* carbuncles; furuncles; furunculosis
Bolotov, A. T., 10
bone fractures, 61, 90
bone pain, 70
Botkin, S. P., 115
boyarinya, 83
breastfeeding. *See* lactation
breathing difficulties , 83, 97, 116, 128
bronchial asthma, 29, 52, 57, 59, 72, 88, 104, 121, 132, 204–205
bronchial catarrh, 88
bronchial problems, 94
bronchiectasis, 35
bronchitis, 34, 57, 59, 62, 63, 64, 70, 72, 75, 77, 79, 80, 91, 94, 97, 104, 106, 110, 117, 119, 128, 134, 140, 141, 143, 199, 202–204 *See also* acute bronchitis; chronic bronchitis
bruises, 31, 112, 128, 142
Bubnov, N. A., 115
buds, 15
bulat, 122

burning flower, 115
burns, 24, 31, 48, 49, 59, 61, 66, 67, 70, 74, 88, 97, 101, 104, 106, 108, 119, 136, 138, 142, 150

calcium, 112
calcium chloride, 149
calculi. *See* bladder stones; gallstones; kidney stones; urolithiasis
callouses, 67
calmative, 28, 35, 52, 67, 69, 74, 88, 94, 102, 104, 110, 113, 116, 134, 135, 145, 148
cancer, 50, 55, 79, 220
carbuncles, 31. *See also* boils; furuncles; furunculosis
cardiac, 31, 48, 99, 106, 113, 116, 143
cardiac arrhythmia, 99, 116, 192–193
cardioactive glycoside, 116
cardioneurosis, 112
cardiosclerosis, 31
cardiovascular insufficiency, 49, 99, 115, 143, 191–192
cardiovascular system, 28, 106, 112, 185–199
carminative, 28, 29, 47, 48, 52, 62, 69, 75, 91, 95, 102, 106, 110, 112, 113, 140, 145, 149
catarrhal diseases, 64, 133. *See also* bladder: bladder catarrh; bronchial catarrh; intestinal catarrh; lung catarrh; stomach: stomach catarrh; throat catarrh; urinary catarrh
catarrhal gastritis, 81
cathartic, 55
caustic, 50
Celts, 126
central nervous system, 28, 31, 35–36, 115, 116
chaga, 55, 56
chapped skin, 25, 117, 142
chemical poisoning, 98
chemotherapy, 55
chest congestion, 137
chest herb, 135
chest pain, 57, 83, 134
children's disorders, 54, 58, 96, 100, 103, 110, 112, 141, 112
Chinese herbal use, 9, 10, 62, 97, 114, 134
chistotel, 50
cholagogue, 28, 31, 32, 35, 41, 44, 50, 62, 67, 72, 81, 88, 89, 100, 104, 106, 112, 113, 134, 146, 149
cholesterol, 58, 77, 83, 98, 106, 146
cholecystitis, 49, 139. *See also* gallbladder
cholelithiasis. *See* gallstones
chromium, 36
chronic bronchitis, 61, 77, 88, 102, 203–204

chronic cholecystitis, 48, 175–176
chronic gastritis, 52, 119, 155–159
chronic glomerulonephritis, 179–180
chronic hepatitis, 32, 172–174
chronic pyelonephritis, 181–182
cirrhosis, 174–175
Clavac tribe, 7
coagulant, 86, 122, 149
colds, 31, 34, 42, 48, 57, 80, 94, 100, 102, 104, 113, 120, 121, 134, 141, 143, 200–202
cold sores, 24
colic, 30, 44, 75, 106, 113, 121, 128
colitis, 32, 34, 77, 79, 90, 142, 148, 162, 165–168
collagenosis, 34
collecting herbs, 13–16
complex herbal formulas, 152: preparing, 18–20
conjunctivitis, 69, 75, 86
constipation, 35, 41, 43, 49, 53, 64, 65, 68, 71, 77, 88, 97, 102, 106, 142, 143
constipation and myocardosis, 189–190
Corglickon, 99
corns, 50, 67, 80
coughs, 34, 42, 57, 59, 63, 65, 69, 75, 80, 100, 103, 104, 106, 110, 117, 121, 136, 141
crawfish's neck, 40
cuts, 24, 43, 46, 48, 49, 119, 133. *See also* wounds
cystitis, 35, 48, 91, 106
cystopyelitis, 104

dandruff, 39, 107, 141
deafness, 90
decoctions, 18
demulcent, 26, 34, 59, 77, 88, 110, 143, 148
deodorizer, 91, 102, 103
depression, 96
depurative, 32, 67, 79, 106, 114, 143, 146
dermatitis, 34, 54, 58, 70, 211–213
dermatomycosis, 74
desire disorders, 228
diabetes mellitus, 34, 44, 49, 54, 57, 70, 74, 94, 97, 106, 107, 112, 120, 133, 136, 144, 170–171
diallyl disulfide, 79
diaphoretic, 28, 31, 32, 38, 44, 50, 52, 67, 70, 79, 93, 95, 102, 104, 112, 120, 146, 149
diarrhea, 29, 34, 37, 40, 53, 59, 72, 74, 88, 90, 94, 106, 109, 114, 115, 119, 120, 121, 128, 136, 140, 141, 142
Diascorides, 8, 46, 75, 92
diathesis, 143
digestive, 28, 29, 35, 41, 62, 72, 77, 91, 95, 106, 135
digestive aid, 52, 53, 61, 65, 72, 79, 81, 90, 91, 113, 119, 128, 136, 141

digestive disorders, 24, 26–27, 29, 31, 35, 46, 52, 79, 81, 84, 94, 106, 141, 143
disbolism, 133
disinfectant, 36, 38, 81, 100, 108, 112, 117, 119, 140
diuretic, 28, 29, 32, 34, 36, 38, 40, 44, 47, 48, 50, 53, 54, 62, 63, 65, 67, 69, 70, 72, 74, 75, 79, 86, 89, 91, 93, 97, 99, 104, 106, 110, 112, 116, 117, 120, 122, 190–191, 132, 134, 135, 143, 146
diverticulitis, 146
dizziness, 83, 96
dodekateon, 63
douche. *See* vaginal douche
dropsy, 65, 94
Druids, 108, 126
drying herbs, 13–16
duodenal ulcers, 32, 52, 73, 74, 77, 88, 97, 104, 119, 133, 142, 150, 159–162
dye, 57, 83
dysentery, 37, 40, 53, 54, 61, 104, 109, 110, 142
dyspepsia, 68, 97, 112, 113, 142
dyskinesia, 163–164

ear, 57, 70, 148
eczema, 32, 37, 39, 44, 45, 52, 54, 57, 62, 67, 70, 74, 75, 90, 97, 103, 106, 108, 110, 114, 120, 122, 133, 136, 142, 211–213
edema, 46, 64, 65, 67, 71, 75, 86, 112, 116
Egyptian herbal use, 29
elixir of life, 66
emaciation, 57
emetic, 70
emmenagogue, 53, 72, 95, 102, 106, 112
emollient, 24, 26, 31, 44, 46, 59, 77, 88, 99
emphysema, 142
endocarditis, 31
endocrine system, 98
enema, 37
enteral syndrome, 164–165
enteritis, 142
enterocolitis, 27, 77, 79, 162
epilepsy, 28, 31, 72, 99, 103, 134, 145
ether oil, 91
eugenol, 95–96
European herbal use, 26, 30, 35, 42, 68, 124–125, 126, 127, 132, 137
expectorant, 26, 28, 29, 35, 59, 60, 61, 62, 64, 72, 75, 84, 89, 91, 97, 100, 102, 106, 110, 113, 117, 119, 136, 137, 140
eye ailments, 69, 99, 137, 141
eye ointment, 70
eyesight, 112
eyewash, 27, 52, 57, 69, 86, 90, 128
face wash, 101

fatigue, 48
fear, 226
febrifuge, 41, 63, 81, 106
Fedorovich, Czar Michael, 72
female reproductive system, 207–210. *See also* lactation; menopause; menstrual cycle; pregnancy
fever, 99, 120, 121, 128
fibroid tumor, 58
fibromyalgia, 217
Filatov, V. P., 24
First World War, 132
fistulas, 105
Flamin, 139
flatulence, 29, 48, 75, 91, 94, 102, 113, 150
flowers, 14
flu. *See* influenza
folk-herbal tradition, 8, 10
food, 2
food poisoning, 77, 98
foot bath, 81
freckles, 65, 66, 112
frostbite, 24, 31, 108
fungal infections, 46, 50, 114, 136, 141
furuncles, 31, 58, 67, 70, 77, 86, 94, 103, 117. See *also* boils; carbuncles
furunculosis, 34, 106, 111, 150

galactagogue, 29, 48, 69, 75, 106
Galen, 8, 75
gallbladder, 175–177: disorders of, 32, 52, 67, 77, 106, 133; improve function of, 79, 139; infections of, 50, 90; inflammation of, 49, 54, 85, 113, 139. *See also* bile
gallstones, 32, 44, 46, 49, 50, 67, 78, 90, 97, 113, 136, 139, 150, 176–177
gargle, 27, 86, 87, 93, 94, 96, 100, 103, 108, 110, 113–114, 115, 119, 130, 141
Gartman's mixture, 140
gastric hypoacidity, 113, 128
gastric spasms, 113
gastritis, 27, 35, 41, 43, 44, 52, 61, 69, 74, 77, 90, 102, 107, 133, 139, 148, 150. *See also* acute gastritis; chronic gastritis
gastrointestinal tract: disorders of, 49, 72, 106, 120, 142, 143; improve function of, 32, 81, 88; inflammation of, 77, 110, 128; spasms of, 53. *See also* intestinal tract; stomach
gastrorrhagia, 132, 168
genital itching, 136
Gentius, King, 81
Georgia, 8
Gerard, John, 103
germifuge, 86
gestational toxicosis, 97, 133

giddiness, 72, 128
gingivitis, 40, 52, 103, 108. *See also* gums; periodontitis
glomerulonephritis, 178–180
Gmelin, Georgovich, 10
goiter, 54, 73, 90
gout, 52, 68, 70, 90, 96, 110, 136, 137. *See also* podagra
Greek herbal use, 8, 26, 46, 63, 75, 81, 92, 111, 113, 114, 127, 132, 149
Grieve, Margaret, 125
Groter, D., 123
gums: bleeding of, 54, 108, 142; disorders of, 90, 103, 138; inflammation of, 96, 112. *See also* gingivitis; periodontitis

hair: coloring, 58; conditioner, 25; graying, 58, 107, 121; growth, 39; loss, 34, 44, 57, 74, 103, 107, 121, 150; rinse, 52, 53; shampoo, 141
halitosis, 112, 113
hay fever, 70
headache, 59, 63, 72, 74, 93, 100, 103, 106, 117, 119, 128, 134, 136, 137, 141, 148. *See also* migraine headache
heart: diseases of, 64, 86, 113, 115; improve function of, 46, 65, 79, 107, 110; palpitations of, 72, 74, 128; spasms of, 127–128. *See also* cardiac; cardiac arrhythmia; cardiosclerosis; cardiovascular insufficiency; cardiovascular system; stenocardia
heartburn, 37, 81
heart rate, 95, 133, 134
hemorrhage, 67, 93, 106, 132, 149
hemorrhoids, 34, 43, 44, 49, 52, 54, 61, 72, 84, 85, 93, 101, 114, 133, 137, 197–199: bleeding of, 37, 86, 149
hemostatic, 31, 32, 35, 36, 53, 60, 72, 74, 84, 89, 104, 106, 108, 119, 120, 132, 134, 135, 142, 149
hepacholecystitis, 32
hepatic, 32, 48
hepaticholecystitis, 139
hepatitis, 172, 139. *See also* chronic hepatitis
herbal baths, 93, 102–103, 108, 109, 141, 215–216
Herbal Book, The, 106
Herbal Institute of the Uzbekistan Academy, 3, 11
herbal juices, 21
herbal medicine, history of, 7–8
herbal research institutes, 3, 11
herb of a thousand leaves, 149
herb of grace, 127
herbs: adverse reactions to, 4; collecting and drying, 13–16; special properties of, 2, 11–12

Herbs of Siberia Used for Cardiovascular Disease, 61
hernia, 94
hiccoughs, 148
high blood pressure. *See* blood pressure
Hippocrates, 8, 75, 127
hives, 52, 97
HIV infection, 87
hoarseness, 75, 136
Hoffman, David, 71
huantesin, 134
hydragogue, 50, 75
hypercelatosis, 58
hyperkeratosis, 121
hypertension, 74, 83, 104, 114, 133, 134
hypertonia, 69, 97
hypnotic, 145
hypochondria, 67
hypotonia, 193–195
hysteria, 28, 104, 113, 145, 225–226

ichthyosis erythroderma, 34
IHD. *See* ischemic heart disease
immortalizer, the, 73, 139
immune stimulator, 39, 52, 81, 87, 106, 220, 221–222
immune system, 219–223
Imperial Academy of Science, 42
indigestion. *See* digestion disorders
influenza, 31, 64, 80, 100, 102, 104, 113, 116, 120, 121, 134, 200–202
infusions, 17–18
Inozemtev, F. I., 99
insect bites, 24, 59, 92–93, 105, 112, 119
insomnia, 28, 52, 53, 63, 67, 69, 74, 80, 96, 102, 113, 134, 136, 137, 141, 145, 148, 224–225
intestinal catarrh, 142
intestinal colic, 41, 136, 146
intestinal gas. *See* flatulence
intestinal peristalsis, 102
intestinal regulator, 77
intestinal tract, 55, 61: bleeding of, 74, 106, 168–169; cramps of, 53; disorders of, 31, 34, 37, 55, 79, 136, 137, 148, 162–168; inflammation of, 61, 106, 109, 121; infections of, 75; irritation of, 163; spasms of, 128, 145; tone of, 132
intestinal worms, 28, 34, 37, 48, 49, 62, 72, 79, 128, 139
intoxication, 120
iridocyclitis, 69
iritis, 69
iron, 36, 67, 112
ischemic heart disease, 187–188
itching, 37, 44, 73, 90, 110, 115, 128, 136,

141, 215–216
Ivan and Maria, 110
Ivan's tea, 147

jaundice, 27, 32, 34, 58, 142. *See also* chronic hepatitis; hepatitis
joint disorders, 52, 62, 63, 68, 78, 85, 90, 96, 104, 110, 141. *See also* arthritis; gout; osteoarthritis; podagra; rheumatism; rheumatoid arthritis
juices, herbal, 21

Kaporic tea, 147
Karl the Great, 26
Kaznacheev, S. B., 61
kidney beans, 170–171
kidneys, 178–184: disorders of, 36, 52, 54, 57, 59, 64, 67, 70, 71, 77, 86, 91, 94, 97, 100, 106, 112, 133, 137; improve function of, 49, 107; infections of, 90; inflammation of, 34, 38, 44, 104, 116, 139, 143
kidney stones, 27, 34, 38, 44, 46, 66, 91, 110, 122, 128, 136, 150
Kiev State Institute for Advanced Medical Training, 50
knight's milfoil, 149
knit-together herb, 60
knowledgists, 9, 55
Kovaliova, N., 25
Krasnoborov, I. M., 61
Kravlov, N. P., 93
Kudryash, 104

lactation, 30, 49, 69, 75, 106, 150
laryngitis, 52, 93, 94, 141, 142
laryngorragia, 132
laxative, 24–25, 32, 41, 48, 53, 60, 71, 77, 97, 99, 110
lead poisoning, 79
leaves, 14
Lepehin, Ivan Ivanovich, 10
leukorrhea, 37, 121
lichen planus, 34, 213–214, 216
Linetol, 77
Linney, K., 123
linseed oil, 77
liver, 172–175: disorders of, 36, 42, 46, 54, 62, 67, 94, 106, 112, 116, 133, 134, 139, 143; improve function of, 29–30, 49, 79, 107, 139; infection of, 90. *See also* bile
lopuh, 44
lumbago, 52
lung catarrh, 85, 94
lungs, 94, 120, 121, 137. *See also* respiratory system
lupus erythematosus, 97

macrophages, 219
magnesium, 112
malaria, 57, 66, 81, 90, 106
massage oil, 77, 78
mastitis, 34
Mattiolus, 92–93
measles, 120
menopause, 209–210
menorrhagia, 207–208. *See also* metrorrhagia; uterine hemorrhage
menstrual cycle, 207: decrease flow, 54, 86, 94, 114; promote onset, 57, 128, 142; regulate, 75, 99, 106, 112
menstrual pain, 30, 46, 52, 54, 57, 72, 86, 96, 102, 106, 113, 132, 145, 209
metabolism, 83
meteroism, 41, 52, 62, 75, 96, 106, 150, 164
metrorrhagia, 57, 85, 114. *See also* menorrhagia; uterine hemorrhage
Michael I, Czar, 137
Middle Ages, 35, 38, 42, 127, 132
migraine headache, 30, 35, 63, 80, 113, 145
Military Medicine Academy, 93
miscarriage, 67
Modern Herbal, A, 125
moisturizer, 24
monasteries, 26
morphine addiction, 32
mother and stepmother, 59
mouth: disinfectant of, 140; disorders of, 59, 110, 114, 115, 121; inflammation of, 128
mouth sores, 46, 54, 77, 94, 137, 138, 142. *See also* stomatitis
mouthwash, 52, 90, 94, 100, 103, 108, 142
mucilaginous, 27, 34, 60, 88, 97
mucous membranes, 91, 97
mucus colitis, 165–167
muscles, 75, 78, 85, 129, 145
musculoskeletal system, 217–218
myocarditis, 31, 83
myocardosis, 188–191

Natasha, 50
Native American herbal use, 7–8, 40, 117
nausea, 29, 96, 113, 133
niacin, 112
ninepowers, 72
nephritis, 35, 106, 178
nephrolithiasis, 112
nephrorragia, 132
nervine, 28, 100, 145
nervous excitability, 74
nervous exhaustion, 35
nervousness, 73, 83, 136, 137, 144, 145
nervous spasms, 127

nervous system, 65, 99, 102: disorders of, 50, 52, 54, 128, 134
nervous tension, 63, 69, 100, 102, 128. *See also* hypertension
neuralgia, 52, 85, 141, 146
neurasthenia, 121
neuritis, 52, 121
neurodermatitis, 32, 52, 52, 67, 75, 90, 106, 142, 211–213
neurosis, 63, 96, 104, 134, 226–228
Nevsky, Prince Alexander, 44
Nosal, I. M., 94
Nosal, M. A., 94
nosebleeds, 94, 106, 115, 132, 149
nose inflammation, 148
nutrient, 34

obesity, 54. *See also* weight loss
October Revolution, 10
official herbal tradition, 8
osteoarthritis, 217–218. *See also* arthritis; rheumatism; rheumatoid arthritis
our lady's herb, 140
ovaries, 58

Pallas, Peotr Simonovich, 10
pancreas, 28, 32, 49
Panteliemon the Healer, 66, 144–145
Paracelsus, 92
penicillin, 9
periodontitis, 40, 110
perspiration, 102, 108
Pertusin, 140
Peter's strength, 111
Peter the Great, Czar, 123
petroselenium, 111
petrosila, 111
pharmaceutical drugs, 2, 3, 11, 12
pharyngitis, 115
phlebitis, 59, 60, 85
Physician's Wording, 10
piles. *See* hemorrhoids
pimples, 34, 39
Piorovsky, A. O., 93
pleurisy, 59
plague, 81
Plantaglutcid, 119
pneumonia, 27, 29, 64, 70, 72, 88, 97, 128, 205–206
podagra, 28, 31, 35, 39, 44, 71, 85, 91, 101, 104, 132, 142, 144. *See also* gout
poisoning, 77, 79, 98
polyphenol, 95
Polysporin, 146
pompholyx, 38

Popov, A. P., 45
potassium, 65, 112
pregnancy, 96, 97, 133
prime blossom, 63
prostatitis, 48, 112
prurigo, 52, 121
Przevalsky, N. M., 123
psoriasis, 34, 67, 70, 106, 111, 112, 114, 121, 214–215, 216
psychotherapy, 224, 226
purgative, 24, 32, 43, 50, 65, 70, 75, 77, 88, 106, 110, 119, 134
purifier, 35
pyrrolizidine alkaloid senkirkine, 60

quinsy, 27, 73, 74, 77, 121

radiation burns, 24
rashes, 44, 54, 67, 87, 105, 115, 128, 136, 141
Refreshing Windtown, 111
refrigerant, 81, 120
rejick, 46
relaxation, 141
renal hemorrhage, 106
respiratory system, 200–206, 219: disorders of, 27, 28, 29, 35, 88, 97, 136, 137; infection of, 141; inflammation of, 65, 70, 77, 113, 117, 120, 121
rheumatism, 28, 39, 52, 57, 62, 63, 68, 70, 71, 75, 85, 91, 101, 103, 104, 106, 110, 117, 120, 132, 134, 137, 142, 144
rheumatoid arthritis, 36, 146, 217. See also arthritis; joint disorders; osteoarthritis
rhinorrhagia, 94, 106, 115, 132
rickets, 58, 103, 110
Roman herbal use, 8, 75, 92, 113, 132
roots, 14
rubefacient, 91, 92, 93
Russian baths, 38, 91
Russian herbalism, 2–4, 7, 8–12
Russian Medicine Newspaper, The, 38
Russian penicillin, 79
Russian Red Book, 81

Sagara, King, 65
Saint Anne, 47
salicin, 104
salicylate, 24
salicylic acid, 104
saponin, 146
sclerosis, 120, 132
scrapes, 31. See also cuts; wounds
seborrhea, 70, 121
Second World War, 3, 73, 79
sedative, 28, 31, 35, 46, 63, 102, 113, 114, 134, 145

serpentine, 40
sexual erethism, 102
scabs, 90
scalp vermin, 112
scarlet fever, 116
sciatica, 85
sciatic neuritis, 85
scrofula, 73, 103, 148
scurvy, 117
Shaman Pharmaceuticals, 12
shampoo, 141
sinusitis, 64, 70
sinus problems, 80
Skif tribe, 7
skin, 101, 211–216: disorders of, 24, 31, 34, 39, 40, 42, 44, 49, 50, 64, 66, 67, 70, 74, 77, 102, 108, 112, 117, 119, 121, 122, 136, 150; discoloration of, 39, 67, 112; grafts, 61; infection of, 141; inflammation of, 94; ulcers, 31, 37, 42, 59, 74, 80, 86, 150.
skin erysipelas, 121
skin rashes. See rashes
skin tuberculosis, 150
Slavic herbal use, 63, 75, 132, 140
snakebite, 119
snake's herb, 135
soap, 129
soldier's wound wort, 149
soporific, 63
sores, 66, 74, 88, 90, 93, 104, 108, 128, 137, 143
spleen, 32
State Botanical Garden, 123
stenocardia, 31, 49, 74, 113, 190
stimulant, 29, 47, 48, 72, 75, 79, 91, 120, 132
stomach: acidity, 26–27, 37, 41, 43, 67, 97, 113, 119; bleeding, 132, 168; catarrh, 53, 88; disorders, 31, 34, 37, 54, 55, 57, 81, 88, 112, 136, 137; inflammation, 61, 67, 52, 121; pains, 99, 119; spasms, 46, 113, 145; ulcers, 26–27, 32, 43, 53, 61, 72, 74, 77, 88, 97, 104, 128, 133, 142, 150, 159–162, 119. See also digestive disorders; gastritis; gastrointestinal tract
stomachic, 29, 35, 36, 48, 52, 60, 62, 67, 69, 72, 75, 81, 84, 89, 91, 95, 102, 104, 106, 108, 112, 113, 120, 145
stomatitis, 40, 52, 108, 153–154. See also gingivitis; mouth sores; periodontitis
Stone Age, 77
styptic, 36, 60, 108, 133, 136, 142, 148
sudorific, 28, 32, 63, 72, 97, 100, 110
sunburn, 24, 112, 136
sweet herb, 97
sweetly scented, 102

synthetic drugs. *See* pharmaceutical drugs

Taber's Cyclopedic Medical Dictionary, 228
tachycardia, 72, 74, 128
tannin, 40
thermos bottle, 20
thiamin, 36
throat catarrh, 59
throat disinfectant, 140
throat: disorders of, 49, 97, 108, 121, 142; inflammation of, 128, 148
thrombophlebitis, 85, 196
thrush, 98
Thymol, 140
thymus gland, 219
thyroid gland, 145
tinctures, 20–21
tinnitus, 134
T-lymphocytes, 219
toad's herb, 73
Tokin, B. P., 79
tonic, 28, 29, 31, 32, 34, 38, 41, 46, 52, 55, 67, 72, 81, 88, 89, 91, 97, 102, 104, 106, 120, 135, 140, 143, 149
tonsillitis, 37, 40, 46, 52, 64, 73, 74, 100, 103, 104, 121, 141
toothache, 54, 70, 93, 103, 110, 114, 119
tooth extractions, 94
trachea, 110
trench herb, 60
trichomoniasis, 109
trophic ulcers, 31, 74, 104
Tubercle bacillus, 88
tuberculosis, 35, 40, 42, 58, 61, 65, 67, 72, 81, 88, 94, 103, 106, 119, 137, 142, 144
tumors, 34, 58

ulcerative colitis, 165, 167–168
ulcers, 24. *See also* duodenal ulcers; skin: skin ulcers; stomach: stomach ulcers; trophic ulcers
ulcers, of the lower leg, 52.
Unguentum calendula, 46
University of St. Petersburg, 104
University of Tomsk School of Medicine, 134
urethritis, 52, 91
urinary acid diathesis, 38
urinary bladder: disorders of, 31, 32, 34, 35, 38, 46, 42, 53, 62, 64, 67, 91, 97, 106; inflammation of, 57, 90, 104, 109, 143
urinary catarrh, 59, 122
urinary tract, 178–184: disorders of, 34, 48, 91, 109, 110, 112, 147; infections of, 32; inflammation of, 86, 143
urinary tract stones. *See* urolithiasis

urination, 27, 104, 112, 137, 139
urolithiasis, 30, 49, 106, 143, 182–184
uterine abrasions, 74
uterine hemorrhage, 25, 31, 52, 54, 57, 74, 85, 93, 106, 112, 114, 149. *See also* menorrhagia
uterine toner, 50, 132, 149–150

vaginal disorders, 109, 143
vaginal douche, 37, 52, 77, 88, 94, 109
vaginitis, 74
vahta, 41
varicose veins, 85, 195
vasculitis, 57, 90, 106, 112, 133, 142
vasoconstrictor, 84, 132
vasodilator, 31, 32, 74, 79, 95, 99, 114, 146
veneral disease, 40
vermicide, 36, 62, 79, 86
vertigo, 30
Virgin Mary, 47, 140
virucidal, 79
vision. *See* eyesight
vitamin deficiency, 106
vitamins: A vitamin, 36, 67, 112, 220; B vitamins, 67, 220; C vitamin, 36, 63, 67, 99, 106, 112, 117, 200, 220; E vitamin, 77, 220
vitiglio, 34, 57, 106, 112, 121
vodka, 20–21
Volhva, 98
vomiting, 55, 81, 96, 113, 120
vulnerary, 24, 31, 35, 36, 46, 50, 53, 60, 70, 72, 74, 77, 86, 88, 89, 102, 104, 106, 114, 120, 137

warts, 50, 67
water banya, 18–20
weight loss, 49, 77
white blood cells, 52, 81
White Snow Maiden, 98
whooping cough, 29, 64, 72, 88, 98, 102, 107, 110, 134, 140, 148
wonderful power, 72
wounds, 24, 31, 39, 42, 44, 46, 48, 52, 54, 58, 61, 70, 74, 81, 90, 94, 96, 103, 105, 106, 115, 119, 133, 136, 138, 141, 142, 148, 150: infected, 49, 80, 86, 93, 117, 143
wrinkles, 24

Xenia of Pskov, Princess, 32

Yagodka, V. C., 50

Zeus, 108
zinc, 220